FIGHTING FIT

FIGHTING FIT

The Israel Defense Forces Guide to Physical Fitness and Self-Defense

Col. DAVID BEN-ASHER

Translated by Miriam Schlesinger

A PERIGEE BOOK

Perigee Books
are published by
The Putnam Publishing Group
200 Madison Avenue
New York, New York 10016

Drawings by Howard Grossman
Photographs by Oded Kirsh and David and Nancy Brown

Library of Congress Cataloging in Publication Data

Ben-Asher, David.
   Fighting fit.

   "A Perigee book."
   1. Physical fitness.   2. Exercise.   3. Self-defense.
4. Israel. Tzeva haganah le-Yiśrael.   I. Title.
[GV481.B44   1983b]   613.7′1   82-402
ISBN 0-399-50624-1 (pbk.)   AACR2

First Perigee printing, 1983

Printed in the United States of America

1 2 3 4 5 6 7 8 9 10

BOOK DESIGN BY BERNARD SCHLEIFER

Acknowledgments

I AM DEEPLY GRATEFUL to all those who contributed to this book for giving their knowledge and themselves over the years to the development of the concepts and methods represented here.

I especially wish to thank:

First Sergeant Major Emi Lichtenfeld and Lieutenant Colonel Shaike Barak for the Contact Combat (*Krav Maga*) section of the book.

Colonel Gidon Snir for the subject of physical fitness and the Obstacles section.

Oded Kirsch, who took the pictures for the Contact Combat section.

The program presented in this book would not have been possible without the contributions of Lieutenant Colonel Giora Kohen; Lieutenant Colonel Amos Bar-Hama; Colonel Eli Yaniv; Lieutenant Colonel Arieh Halevi; Colonel Moshel Zohar; M.D. Colonel Yair Shapirah; Sergeant Major Andra Avigal; Colonel Nir Nitzan; Lieutenant Colonel Avraham Yehezkel; Lieutenant Colonel Menachem Rak-oz; Lieutenant Colonel David Gerstein; Major Amos Golani; Mr. Nadav Shlomo, the writer.

M.D. Oded Bar-or; Dr. Gilad Wingarten; Dr. Omri Imbar; Dr. Dov Aldubi; Dr. Alberto Aa'yalon; Dr. Mosheh Katz; Mr. Arieh Rosentzwig; Dr. Hilel Ruskin; Dr. Uri Zimri; Mr. Uri Afek; Mr. Yariv Oren; Mr. Shalom Hermon; M.D. Professor Ezra Zohar; M.D. Yehuda Sheinfeld; Dr. David Eldar; Dr. Michael Hertzig; Professor Ema Giron; Dr. Elimelech Shochat; Dr. Micha Kanitz.

I also wish to thank the following for their invaluable assistance in the preparation of this book: Gidon Shamir; Peter Halban; Lt. Col. Giora Cohen; Matti Steiner; Sgt. Major Eli Avigzar; Lauren Gelper; Miriam Schlesinger for her translation of original material; and Michele Salcedo.

—COL. DAVID BEN-ASHER

To the memory of my parents
Hannah and Benjamin Ben-Asher

Contents

PART II   SELF-DEFENSE—CONTACT COMBAT

PART III.   OBSTACLES

PART IV.   PHYSIOLOGICAL ASPECTS
OF PHYSICAL EFFORT

Foreword

A FIGHTING ARMY MUST have outstanding endurance and skill. Its soldiers must overcome obstacles in the field and in cities, succeed in hand-to-hand combat with or without a weapon, get through water obstacles, move correctly, and advance swiftly and effectively. The Israel Defense Forces (I.D.F.) devotes a great deal of effort toward making its fighting men and women the best in the world. Toward that goal, they have three major objectives:

1. professional competence;
2. high morale and fighting spirit; and
3. physical development and motor abilities are stressed in each training segment, beginning with the physical fitness program.

Men and women between the ages of 18 and 55 make up the I.D.F. The physical training program has, therefore, been adapted to the diversity of the soldiers as well as to the needs of all the different branches of the Israeli military and includes a broad range of methods and activities. We have developed precise criteria for measuring results. Supervision and follow-up procedures enable us to keep track of our soldiers' achievements and long-term development. These different methods form an integrated strategy to promote interest in physical activity, intensify motivation, and minimize the dangers of overexertion.

This book provides a systematic presentation of the combat fitness program used by the I.D.F. It is divided into clearly outlined sections, each with a specific goal. Everything in this book is military in character, but can easily be applied to civilian life, for both groups or individuals. In compiling the material for this book and writing the inter-explanatory material, I have tried to set forth a variety of topics. The reader may choose those that particularly interest him or her to develop a personalized fitness training program.

—COL. DAVID BEN-ASHER

PART I

Physical Fitness

General Physical Fitness

PHYSICAL FITNESS has steadily gained popularity in recent years. Advocates have embroidered the old slogans—"Run for your health," "A sound mind in a sound body," "Those who do not find time for exercise will have to find time for illness"—into new ones. Thousands are now talking about fitness, a subject that was virtually unmentioned a few years ago.

Talk eventually leads to thought (would that the order were reversed) and soon the brain commands legs, arms and other neglected parts of our bodies. Suddenly, people try to get their bones moving out of the blasé passivity that has been with them for years or even decades. "And the bones came together, bone to his bone . . . the sinews and the flesh came upon them . . ." and the prophecy of Ezekial comes true, causing hearts to pound.

Let's say a person is about to take the fateful plunge, spring out of bed one bright morning and feel his body tingle with youthful vim. He finds himself faced with a dizzying choice. Unless there is a plan that takes into account one's current physical condition, and outlines specific goals so that progress is perceived, the efforts are all too often abandoned. The number of fitness programs a person has to choose from is staggering. There are thousands of programs offered through health clubs and fitness centers, through local Y's and extension programs, there are private dance, exercise and movement groups and, of course, a wide variety of sports to choose from. Many systems have been worked out all over the world for developing physical fitness—some of them ultra-scientific, others less so—each with the backing of some well-known personality.

The Israel Defense Forces System

The I.D.F. combat fitness program is geared toward achieving high fitness levels in the shortest time through strenuous physical exercise.

The I.D.F. system is based on two principles:

A. Testing to measure performance and establish fitness levels (indexes).
B. Combining these indexes to produce an integrated and thorough exercise program.

The indexes are based on data drawn from tests and follow-up studies over the years on hundreds of thousands of soldiers, both men and women. The tables in this chapter represent levels of achievement and provide goals for a continuing fitness program.

Before you begin any fitness program, consult your doctor. Have a thorough physical examination, including an EKG, and discuss your plans to take up a fitness program with him or her. He or she will advise you of any restrictions that may be necessary.

Physical Fitness and Its Components

PHYSICAL FITNESS refers to the ability to perform day-to-day activities "efficiently." In a well-rounded program, specific activities develop specific components of physical fitness. The I.D.F. program concentrates on endurance, flexibility, strength and speed.

Endurance is the ability to persevere at an activity involving exertion, where several groups of muscles are activated, for as long as possible (long-distance swimming, long-distance running). Of all the components, endurance is the most important. It affects all the others.

Strength is the ability to apply maximum muscular exertion (lifting 100 pounds).

Speed is the ability to perform the greatest number of repeated movements in the shortest time.

Other related components:

Power is the ability to overcome great resistance using one's muscles over a length of time (50 push-ups).

Quickness (agility) is the ability to change one's body position in the shortest possible time (change directions while running).

Flexibility is the ability to move one's limbs with ease and agility; to be supple (bending until one's head touches one's knees).

Coordination is the ability to direct and control parts of the body (riding a bicycle).

Accuracy is the ability to control performance vis-à-vis an external object (marksmanship).

Some also include the following as physical fitness components:

Health is the ability to resist disease and injury. None of the components mentioned above can be achieved if the athlete is not in good health.

Motivation is the desire to achieve a goal. It is unlikely that any athlete can do well without motivation.

The Principles of Physical Fitness Training

A. *Resistance*—There must be a certain amount of resistance in the exercise to develop or maintain muscular strength. The level of resistance should be gradually increased by performing the exercise more rapidly.

B. *Graduated Exercising*—Begin with a light exercise load and increase slowly to the highest level of difficulty.

C. *Perseverance*—A high level of physical fitness can be attained by training at least three times a week. This is the best way to keep in shape over a long period. As soon as training stops, physical fitness declines. If the interruption of training is extensive, there is liable to be a steep decline in fitness.

D. *Variety*—The range of physical activities should be varied to maintain interest.

E. *Amount*—The choice of the initial level of resistance always depends on the training method, which, in turn, depends on the current fitness level of the particular athlete. A shot-putter, for example, will train differently than a basketball player.

Three Safety Rules of Physical Fitness

1. Avoid strenuous activity during the hottest hours of the day.
2. When exercising, don't forget to exhale during exertion.
3. Avoid sudden exertion. Let the body adjust to stress *gradually*.

General Military Fitness Tests for Men and Women

THIS TEST IS GIVEN to all soldiers, youth and reserve soldiers up to 54 years of age, and is based on athletic as well as military elements, emphasizing endurance and strength. Israeli soldiers must be in the finest physical condition of all members of the I.D.F., therefore this test is difficult. The established criteria require soldiers to wear military uniforms and army shoes. Nonetheless, the average soldier who wears gym clothes and scores well may be considered in good physical condition.

Although scores of 67 points for men and 75 points for women are considered excellent, the Israeli soldier strives for a perfect score. Generally, the higher the score, the better the soldier.

Because the general military fitness test is so strenuous, be sure to consult your doctor before you take it.

Instructions for Taking the Test

1. Clothing: Full combat uniform, army shoes; or denims or gym clothes, army shoes or jogging shoes.
2. An 8- to 15-minute warm-up prior to the test is mandatory. Duration of warm-up depends on such conditions as temperature, humidity, fatigue from previous activity, as well as your level of fitness. Those who are fit will need less time to warm up. Indications of sufficient warm-up: a very light sweat; muscles feel loosened. For warm-up exercises, see pages 24 and 34.
3. The test is taken as an uninterrupted sequence. The 2,000 meter run comes last.
4. Age-group C, men, 36 years and over, is tested on the 2,000 meter run only; women, 31 years years and over, 1,000 meter run only.

General Military Fitness Test for Men

1. Sit-ups
   A. The test is carried out in pairs.
   B. Lie on a flat surface, with knees bent 90 degrees, feet flat on the floor, 12 inches apart, and hands behind neck. Have the partner hold your feet down so that heels and feet are touching the floor throughout.
   C. Perform as many sit-ups as possible in thirty seconds, with elbows touching knees in sitting position and shoulders touching the floor in supine position.
2. Pull-ups.
   A. Grasp the bar with palms facing forward (thumbs towards one another), and bend elbows until chin clears the bar. Body or legs should not swing. In suspended position, arms and legs are fully extended, feet clear of the floor.
   B. The score is determined by counting each complete pull-up.
   C. Stop counting when you stop exercising for two seconds or more or when chin fails to clear the bar.
3. 2,000 meter run
   A. The track must be flat and solid (hard-packed sand, cinders, asphalt, etc.). It may be either straight or round, with a circumference of no less than 200 meters. Then start and finish should be clearly marked. If a track is not used, the course should be well defined.
   B. Start and timing are in compliance with established procedures for long distance running.
   C. Results are measured in minutes and seconds.

SCORES AND RESULTS

Score Chart
(total points)

Grade/Age	Very good	Good	Pass	Fail
Age-group A: 17 to 25 years	67 and over	56–66	37–55	Below 37
Age-group B: 26 to 35 years	60 and over	50–59	33–49	Below 33
Age-group C (2000 meter run only): 36 years and over	08:30 and below	08:31–10:00	10:01–14:00	Over 14:00

Score **Exercise**

	Sit-ups	Pull-ups	2,000 M run
1	16	1	16.37–17.15
2	17	2	16.02–16.36
3	18		15.30–16.01
4	19	3	14.59–15.29
5	20		14.29–14.58
6	21	4	14.02–14.28
7	22		13.36–14.01
8	23	5	13.10–13.35
9	24	6	12.45–13.09
10	25	7	12.22–12.44
11	26	8–9	12.00–12.21
12	27	10–11	11.39–11.59
13	28	12–15	11.18–11.38
14	29	16–19	10.58–11.17
15	30	20 and over	10.39–10.57
16	31		10.21–10.38
17	32		10.02–10.20
18	33–34		9.50–10.01
19	35–36		9.35–9.49
20	37 and over		9.21–9.34
21			9.07–9.20
22			8.84–9.06
23			8.42–8.83
24			8.31–8.41
25			8.20–8.30
26			8.10–8.19
27			8.00–8.09
28			7.51–7.59
29			7.42–7.50
30			7.34–7.41
31			7.26–7.33
32			7.19–7.25
33			7.12–7.18
34			7.06–7.11
35			7.00–7.05
36			6.55–6.59
37			6.50–6.54
38			6.46–6.49
39			6.45 and below
40			

General Military Fitness Test For Women

1. Sit-ups
   A. The test is carried out in pairs.
   B. Lie on a flat surface, with knees bent about 90 degrees, feet flat on the floor, 12 inches apart, and hands behind neck. Have the partner hold your feet down so that heels and feet are touching the floor throughout.
   C. Perform as many sit-ups as you can in one minute, with elbows touching knees in sitting position and shoulders touching the floor in supine position.
2. Raising arms with weight
   A. Stand erect holding in both hands a rifle, or a bar weight of 6 to 7 pounds, at chest height. Straighten elbows in a gradual uninterrupted movement until rifle or weight is over head. Return to starting position.
   B. Perform the exercise as many times as you can in 90 seconds.
3. 1,000 meter run
   A. The track must be flat and solid (hard-packed sand, cinders, asphalt, etc.). It may be either straight or round, with a circumference of no less than 200 meters. The start and finish should be clearly marked. If a track is not used, the course should be well defined.
   B. Results are measured in minutes and seconds.

SCORES AND RESULTS

Score Chart
(total points)

Grade/Age	Very good	Good	Pass	Fail
Age-group A: 16 to 24 years	75 and over	65–74	50–64	Below 50
Age-group B: 25 to 30 years	56 and over	45–55	35–44	Below 35
Age-group C (1,000 meter run only): 31 years and over	5:30 and below	05:30–06:30	06:31–08:00	Over 8:00

Score	Sit-ups	Raising arms with weight	1,000 M run
Score		**Exercise**	
0	14 and below	43 and below	8:16 and above
1	15–16	44–47	8:11–8:15
2	17–18	48–51	8:06–8:10
3		52–55	8:01–8:05
4	19–20	56–59	7:56–8:00
5		60–63	7:51–7:55
6	21–22	64–67	7:46–7:50
7		68–71	7:41–7:45
8	23–24	72–75	7:36–7:40
9		76–79	7:31–7:35
10	25–26	81–83	7:26–7:30
11	27–28	84–87	7:21–7:25
12	29–30	88–91	7:16–7:20
13	31–32	92–95	7:11–7:15
14	33–34	96–99	7:06–7:10
15	35–36	100–103	7:01–7:05
16	37–38	104–107	6:56–7:00
17	39–40	108–111	6:51–6:55
18	41–42	112–115	6:46–6:50
19	43–44	116–119	6:41–6:45
20	45–46	120 and above	6:36–6:40
21	47–48		6:31–6:35
22	49–50		6:26–6:30
23	51–52		6:21–6:25
24	53–54		6:16–6:20
25	55–56		6:11–6:15
26	57–58		6:06–6:10
27	59–60		6:01–6:05
28	61–62		5:56–6:00
29	63–64		5:51–5:55
30	65 and above		5:46–5:50
31			5:41–5:45
32			5:36–5:40
33			5:31–5:35
34			5:26–5:30
35			5:21–5:25
36			5:16–5:20
37			5:11–5:15
38			5:06–5:10
39			5:01–5:05
40			4:56–5:00
41			4:51–4:55
42			4:46–4:50
43			4:41–4:45
44			4:36–4:40

Exercise

Score	Sit-ups	Raising arms with weight	1,000 M run
45			4:31–4:35
46			4:26–4:30
47			4:21–4:25
48			4:16–4:20
49			4:11–4:15
50			4:10 and below

Mile Fitness Program (M.F.P.)

MEN AND WOMEN can achieve a high level of fitness within four to twelve weeks with this simple and varied program. The Mile Fitness Program (M.F.P.) combines running and calisthenics at specific intervals to develop four of the major components of physical fitness—flexibility, endurance, strength and power—throughout the body in just 15 minutes a day.

Equipment Needed: Gym clothes and sneakers; digital watch, a watch with a second hand, or a stopwatch.

Area: Any level area, with six 220-yard intervals and one 440-yard interval marked off.

Points to Emphasize:

1. Before you begin the M.F.P., have a thorough physical examination. Discuss the program with your doctor. His or her advice will help you avoid injuries.
2. During the breaks, make sure your pulse slows to 120 beats per minute before beginning the next interval. Twenty seconds is the optimum time for your pulse to slow down. In the beginning, it may take longer.
3. Start slowly. The times given for each interval and the maximum number of repeats for the exercises are for higher physical fitness levels. Begin by performing as much of the program as you can in 15 minutes, and gradually work up to the optimum times and repeats on the chart.

4. Maintain a high level of fitness by performing the program two or three times a week.

The Program

WARM-UP:

Interval I

1. Run 440 yards at a light pace. (3 minutes)

2. Flexibility Exercises.

   A. Stand straight, feet apart, arms out to sides at shoulder height. Bend forward from the waist, bring arms together and touch the ground, bending knees slightly if necessary. Return to starting position. (Repeat exercise as many times as possible at a moderate pace within 40 seconds).

   B. Stand straight, feet apart, arms out to sides at shoulder height. Swing right arm across chest and turn trunk to the left as far as possible. Swing arms and trunk to the right as far as possible. (Repeat exercise as many times as possible at a moderate pace within 40 seconds.)

   C. Stand straight, feet apart, arms down at sides. Raise right arm over head and to the left, bending trunk up and over from the waist as far as possible. Return to starting position. Raise left arm overhead and to the right, bending trunk as far as possible. Return to starting position. (Repeat exercise as many times as possible at a moderate pace within 40 seconds.)

POWER BUILDING:

Interval II

1. Run 220 yards at a fast pace. (40 seconds)

2. Break: Walk in a circle. Check your pulse. When the rate drops to 120 beats per minute, go on to step 3. (20 seconds)

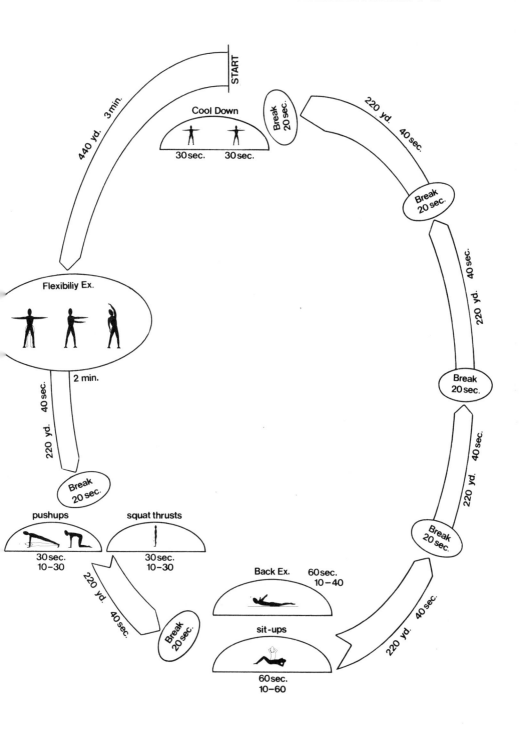

3. Calisthenics:

A. Push-ups: Men perform four-point push-ups; women, six-point push-ups. (Begin with ten and work up to thirty within 30 seconds.)

B. Squat-thrusts: Stand straight, feet together, arms down at sides. Bend knees and squat down, hands on ground in front. Kick legs back into front-support position. (In the front-support position, weight is supported on hands and toes; it's the starting position for a push-up.) Jump back into squat. Return to starting position. (Begin with ten and work up to thirty within 30 seconds.)

Interval III

1. Run 220 yards at a fast pace. (40 seconds)

2. Break: Walk in a circle. Check your pulse. When the rate drops to 120 beats per minute, go on to step 3. (20 seconds)

3. Calisthenics:

A. Sit-ups: Lie on back, hands behind head, knees bent. Raise trunk until elbows touch knees. Return to starting position. (Begin with ten and work up to sixty within 60 seconds.)

B. Back exercise: Lie on stomach, arms extended forward. Raise arms, trunk and legs simultaneously. Return to starting position. (Begin with ten and work up to forty within 60 seconds.)

ENDURANCE:

Interval IV

1. Run 220 yards at a fast pace. (40 seconds)

2. Break: Walk in a circle. Check your pulse. When the rate drops to 120 beats per minute, go on to Interval V. (20 seconds)

Interval V

1. Run 220 yards at a fast pace. (40 seconds)

2. Break: Walk in a circle. Check your pulse. When the rate drops to 120 beats per minute, go on to Interval VI. (20 seconds)

Interval VI

1. Run 220 yards at a fast pace. (40 seconds)

2. Break: Walk in a circle. Check your pulse. When the rate drops to 120 beats per minute, go on to Interval VII. (20 seconds)

Interval VII

1. Run 220 yards at a fast pace. (40 seconds)

2. Break: Walk in a circle. Check your pulse. When the rate drops to 120 beats per minute, continue the cool-down. (20 seconds)

COOL-DOWN:

1. Stand straight, feet apart, arms out to sides at shoulder height. Bend forward from the waist, bring arms together and touch the ground. Return to starting position. (Continue exercise at an easy pace for 30 seconds.)

2. Stand straight, feet apart, arms out to sides at shoulder height. Swing right arm across chest and turn trunk to the left as far as possible. Swing both arms to the right, turning trunk to the right as far as possible. (Continue exercise at an easy pace for 30 seconds.)

Fitness Test for Youth

THE FOLLOWING IS a self-administered test comprised of three elements and a score chart. Endurance may be tested in one of four ways and arm strength in one of two. Sit-ups and squat-thrusts, however, are mandatory.

Instructions for Taking the Test

1. Clothing: Gym clothes; jogging shoes or sneakers.
2. An 8- to 15-minute warm-up prior to the test is mandatory. Duration of warm-up depends on temperature, humidity, and fatigue from previous activity. Indications of sufficient warm-up: a very light sweat; muscles feel loosened. For warm-up exercises, see pages 24 and 34.
3. The test is taken in an uninterrupted sequence. The endurance element comes last.

The test consists of:

1. *Push-ups*—Lie on your stomach, palms flat on floor on either side of chest, elbows bent. Push against floor, raising body and legs off floor in a straight line, until arms are straight and weight is supported on hands and toes. Bend elbows, keeping body and legs straight, until chest rests on floor.

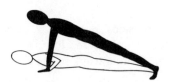

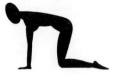

or

Pull-ups—Jump up and grasp bar with palms facing forward (thumbs toward one another), and lift up, bending elbows, until chin clears the bar. Body and legs should not swing. In suspended position, arms and legs are fully extended, feet clear off the floor.

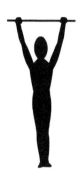 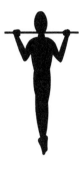

2. *Squat-thrusts*—Bend knees until palms touch the ground, but do not bend knees completely. Move legs straight back; weight is supported on hands and toes. Keep body straight. Bring legs back to squatting position. Stand up.

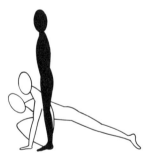

3. *Sit-ups without leg support*—Lie on a flat surface, with knees bent 90 degrees, feet flat on floor, 12 inches apart and hands behind neck. Sit up and touch elbows to knees. Return to starting position.

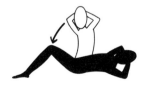

4. *Endurance*—Run for 12 minutes at as quick a pace as you can maintain.

or

Run a 3,000-meter distance.

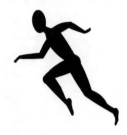

or

Swim a 1,000-meter distance.

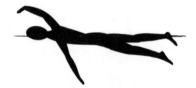

or

Ride a bicycle for 12 minutes at as quick a pace as you can maintain.

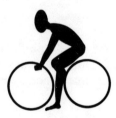

Fitness Test for Youth

The Exercise	Fair	Good	Very Good
Push-ups	20 times	30 times	40 times
or			
Pull-ups (Overhand grasp)	6 times	9 times	12 times
Squat-thrusts	20 times per min.	25 times per min.	30 times per min.
Sit-ups (without leg support)	40 times	50 times	60 times
Running for 12 min.	2,500 m.	2,800 m.	3,000 m.
or			
3,000-m. run	15 min.	13.5 min.	12 min.
or			
Swimming, 1,000 m.	25 min.	22 min.	19 min.
or			
Bicycle riding, 12 min.	5 km.	5.5 km.	6 km.

Methods

NOW THAT YOU KNOW what shape you're in, it's time to get into training. Performing the test exercises everyday will increase your score, but repetition breeds boredom, which soon turns into loss of interest. The program that follows offers varied suggestions for training and exercising that were designed to improve your scores on the various indexes.

Again, there is an abundance and variety of training programs in the world. The trouble is that they tend to be geared to those who are naturally athletic. The more sophisticated the program, the harder it is for the general public to use it efficiently. The obvious danger is the vicious circle, where only those who are already fit can use the available guidance.

The methods presented here, based on the ones used in the I.D.F., will provide a simple but effective approach for anybody interested in improving his or her physical fitness.

The Collective System of Fitness Training—Lesson Plans

IN THE I.D.F. WE usually work in groups rather than individually. Our system incorporates 29 lessons, each lasting 50 minutes. Individuals or pairs can, of course, adapt these group lessons to their own needs. Trainees who perform the entire set of lessons (four to six hours a week) are expected to attain a satisfactory level of physical fitness in six weeks.

The four sample lesson plans given here can be used as models.

Lesson Plan #1

Subject of the lesson: Physical fitness.

Goal: To develop physical ability.

Stages of the lesson and duration of each:

I.	Introduction	10 minutes
II.	400-meter warm-up	3 minutes
III.	Calisthenics	5 minutes
IV.	Strength-building exercises	20 minutes
V.	Soccer game	12 minutes
	Total	50 minutes

SETTING UP THE LESSON

Location: Sandy area, training field.

Instruction methods: Explanation, demonstration and drilling.

Training group: A unit of twenty to forty soldiers.

Preparation for instruction: Inspection of training area and track.

Accessories and equipment: Soccer balls.

Clothing and gear: Military uniform or denims. Gym clothes are preferred; gym shoes or sneakers.

Breakdown of the Lesson

STAGE I: Introducing the Lesson to the Unit—10 Minutes

A. The soldiers sit in rows, backs to the sun.
B. *Opening*—This lesson is designed to improve general physical fitness: strength, power, agility, speed and endurance.

This lesson's requirements are minimal. In subsequent lessons, there will be a gradual increase in the level of difficulty and hence in the soldier's physical fitness.
C. If a soldier fails to complete the series of exercises, he is reminded that the exercises require no more than average ability, and he has not met the grade. If he does succeed, he should be commended and it would be wise to stress that he must have kept in good physical condition before his recruitment.
D. The lesson should be explained stage by stage: running, calisthenics, strength-building exercises and endurance-building exercises.

    1. *Running*—Warm-up speeds up circulation and loosens major muscle groups to prepare the body for greater exertion.
    2. *Calisthenics*—Warm-up specific muscle groups and increase flexibility.
    3. *Strength-building exercises*—Develop muscles. Each exercise is performed in three sets, with a brief rest in between sets, to use each muscle to the fullest.
    4. *Endurance-building exercises*—2,000–3,000-meter run, interval run or a soccer or rugby game.

STAGE II: The 400-Meter Warm-up Run—3 Minutes

A. The unit is arranged in threes, facing the direction it will run.
B. The soldiers sing or clap hands and run in rhythm at a moderate pace.
C. The instructor runs alongside and slightly behind the soldiers.
D. At the end of the run, the soldiers get into rows with their backs to the sun.

STAGE III: Calisthenics—5 Minutes

Before each exercise, the instructor slowly demonstrates the complete movement, counting aloud and emphasizing specific points.

A. *Easy arm exercise—legs apart (count of two, ten times)*

Points to emphasize: Arms are extended and movements are sharp. Warms up arm muscles.

1. At the command "legs apart," soldiers jump into legs-apart position.
2. At the command "exercise at count two, begin," soldiers perform the exercise to the rhythm set by the instructor until the command "and stop."

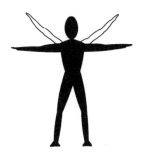

    Count 1 Swing arms back at an angle.
    Count 2 Swing arms forward at an angle.
3. At the command "legs together," soldiers jump into legs-together position.

B. *Forward trunk bends—legs apart, arms raised to the sides (count of four, ten times)*

Points to emphasize: Pelvis is fixed and legs are straight. Increases flexibility.

1. At the command "legs apart," soldiers jump into legs-apart position.
2. At the command "exercise at count four, begin," the soldiers perform the exercise to the rhythm set by the instructor until the command "and stop."
    Count 1 From the waist, bend trunk to the left, to waist-high level.
    Count 2–3 Bounce twice.
    Count 4 Back to upright position.
    Count 1 Bend to right.

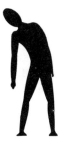

Count 2–3 Bounce twice.
Count 4 Back to upright position.
3. At the command "legs together," soldiers jump into legs-together position.

C. *Sideways trunk turns—legs apart, hands on waist (count of four, six times in each direction)*

Points to emphasize: Lift opposite heel. Increases flexibility.

1. At the command "legs apart," soldiers jump into legs-apart position, hands on waist.
2. At the command "exercise at count four, begin," the soldiers perform the exercise to the rhythm set by the instructor until the command "and stop."

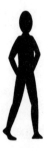

Count 1 Turn trunk to the left, raising heel of opposite leg.
Count 2–3 Bounce twice.
Count 4 Return to starting position.
Count 1 Turn trunk to the right.
Count 2–3 Bounce twice.
Count 4 Return to starting position.
3. At the command "legs together," soldiers jump into legs-together position, arms at sides.

D. *Trunk—legs apart, arms raised to the sides (count of four, eight times)*

Points to emphasize: Keep knees straight; stomach pulled in while stretching arms back. Warm-up; increases flexibility of back.

1. At the command "starting position," soldiers jump into legs-apart position, arms extended at shoulder height.
2. At the command "exercise at count four, begin," the soldiers perform the exercise to the rhythm set by the instructor until the command "and stop."

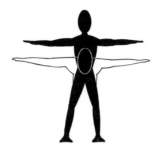

Count 1–2 Stretch arms back and bend trunk forward; bounce once.

Count 3 Return to upright position, stretching arms to the sides at shoulder height.

Count 4 Stretch arms back again.

3. At the command "legs together," soldiers jump into legs-together position.

E. *Difficult arm exercise—front-support or push-up position (count of two, ten times)*

Points to emphasize: Bring chest close to the ground while keeping knees and trunk straight. Correct breathing: inhale while bending arms, exhale when straightening. Strengthens arms.

1. At the command "down to front support at count two," soldiers squat thrust (count 1) to front-support position (count 2) to the rhythm set by the instructor.

2. At the command "exercise at count two, begin," soldiers begin the exercise to the rhythm set by the instructor until the command "and stop."

Count 1 Bend elbows.

Count 2 Straighten elbows.

3. At the command "into upright position at count two," soldiers complete squat thrust (count 1) to upright position (count 2).

STAGE IV: Strength-Building Exercises—20 Minutes

A. *Back—lying facedown, hands crossed on forehead, elbows out (count of two, three rounds of ten times each)*

Points to emphasize: Correct breathing: exhale when rising, inhale when descending. Strengthens back muscles.

1. At the command "face-down position at count three," soldiers get into starting position at the rhythm set by the instructor.

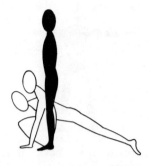

Count 1 Squat, arms between legs, palms flat on ground.
Count 2 Throw legs back into front-support position.
Count 3 Bend elbows, lowering body to ground until forehead rests on hands.

2. At the command "exercise at count two, begin," soldiers perform the exercise ten times at the rhythm set by the instructor until the command "and rest."

Count 1 Raise chest and arms, arching upper back.
Count 2 Lower chest and arms to ground.
Pause between rounds in face-down position, resting on forearms, elbows out.

3. On completing three rounds, at the command "upright at count three," soldiers return to upright position.

Count 1 Palms flat on ground, straighten arms to front-support position.
Count 2 Squat.
Count 3 Rise to upright position.

B. *Arms and chest—front-support position (count of two, three rounds of ten times each)*

Points to emphasize: Knees and trunk must be straight. Breathe correctly: inhale when bending, exhale when straightening. Strengthens arm, back and stomach.

1. At the command "down to front support at count two," soldiers descend to front-support position.
2. At the command "exercise at count two, begin," soldiers perform the exercise ten times at the rhythm set by the instructor, until the command "and rest."

Count 1 Bend elbows until chest touches ground.
Count 2 Straighten elbows, raising trunk off ground.

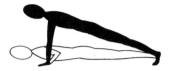

3. At the command "knees down," soldiers lower knees to the ground and rest in the six-point position between rounds. At the command "get set," the soldiers resume starting position.
4. On completing three rounds, at the command "upright on count two," soldiers return to upright position.

C. *Abdomen—lying on back, forearm support (count of two, three rounds of eight times each)*

Points to emphasize: Correct breathing: exhale when raising legs, inhale when lowering them. Strengthens stomach, thighs and hips.

1. At the command "down to back on count two," soldiers get into starting position.
    Count 1 Squat down. Place hands on ground behind back for support.

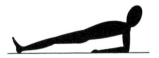

    Count 2 Lean body back and extend legs forward.
2. At the command "exercise at count two, begin," the soldiers perform the exercise eight times at the rhythm set by the instructor, until the command "and rest."
    Count 1 Raise legs, extended, to a 45-degree angle.

    Count 2 Lower legs to ground.
    Rest in starting position.

3. On completing rounds, at the command "upright at count two," soldiers return to upright position.

   Count 1 Sit up and roll forward into squatting position.

   Count 2 Stand up.

D. *Abdomen—lying on back, hands clasped behind head, elbows out to sides (count of two, three rounds of ten times each)*

   Points to emphasize: Back must be straight and erect when sitting. Correct breathing: exhale when rising and inhale when descending. Strengthens stomach, chest and thighs.

   1. At the command "down to back at count two," soldiers get into back position at the rhythm set by the instructor.

      Count 1 Squat down. Place hands on ground behind back for support.

      Count 2 Lean body back until back is resting on ground, hands clasped behind head, elbows out; extend legs forward.

   2. At the command "exercise at count two, begin," soldiers perform the exercise ten times at the rhythm set by the instructor, until the command "and rest."

      Count 1 Rise to sitting position.

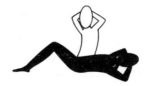

      Count 2 Return to back.

      Rest between rounds on back, with knees bent.

   3. On completing three rounds, at the command "upright at count two," soldiers return to upright position.

      Count 1 Sit up and roll forward into squatting position.

      Count 2 Stand up.

STAGE V: Soccer Game—12 Minutes

A. Game is played in keeping with the rules for soccer.

B. If there are over twenty-five soldiers in the unit, divide into four teams.

Lesson Plan #2

Subject of the lesson: Cyclical drill.

Goal: To develop physical ability.

Stages of the lesson and duration of each:

I.	Introduction	5 minutes
II.	400-meter warm-up run	3 minutes
III.	Calisthenics	5 minutes
IV.	Drilling	32 minutes
V.	Summation	5 minutes
	Total	50 minutes

SETTING UP THE LESSON

Location: Open area.

Instruction methods: Explanation, demonstration and drilling.

Training group: A unit of twenty to forty soldiers.

Preparation for instruction: Inspect training area and decide on location of ten activity points. Set up equipment.

Accessories and equipment (for unit of twenty): Twenty half-kilo medicine balls, marking strips, pail, three crates or benches (two 40 cm. high; one 60 cm. high), two walls (150 cm. high, 150 cm. wide), ropes (4 meters long), whistle.

Clothing and gear: Military uniform, denims or gym clothes; army boots or gym shoes.

BREAKDOWN OF THE LESSON

STAGE I: Introducing the Lesson to the Unit—15 Minutes

A. Soldiers sit in rows, backs to the sun, at the center of the ten activity points.
B. *Opening*—This lesson is designed to improve strength, endurance, power, flexibility and agility. These exercises and the skills they develop can easily be adapted to different terrains and obstacles. This lesson requires a good level of fitness.

C. The lesson should be explained stage by stage:

Running—Reiterate value as warm-up to prepare body for greater exertion by increasing circulation and by loosening large muscle groups.

Calisthenics—Warms up specific muscle groups and increases flexibility.

Drilling—Develops strength, power, flexibility and endurance.
Each exercise is performed at a different point and in a specific order to strengthen and build different muscle groups. The variety of the exercises increases interest in performance. The lesson can be set up as competition between groups to increase motivation even more.

STAGE II: The 400-Meter Warm-Up Run—3 Minutes

A. The unit is arranged in threes, facing the direction it will run.
B. The soldiers sing or clap hands and run in rhythm at a moderate pace.
C. The instructor runs at the end of the line.
D. At the end of the run, the soldiers get into rows with their backs to the sun.

STAGE III: Calisthenics—5 Minutes

Before each new exercise, the instructor slowly demonstrates the complete movement, counting aloud and emphasizing specific points.

A. *Easy arm exercise—legs apart, arms out to the sides at shoulder level (count of four, ten to twelve times)*

Points to emphasize: Pull stomach in. Increases circulation and arm flexibility.

   1. Command: "Legs apart."
   2. Command: "Exercise at count four, begin."
      Count 1–2 Two forward circular arm movements.

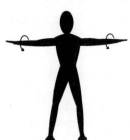

Count 3–4 Two backward circular arm movements.
Command: "And stop."
3. Command: "Legs together."

B. *Back exercise—legs apart, arms extended upwards (count of four, fifteen times)*

Points to emphasize: Turn slowly and bend fully in each direction. Increases flexibility.

    1. Command: "Legs apart."
    2. Command: "Exercise at count four, begin."
        Count 1–2 Two trunk turns from right to left.
        Count 3–4 Two trunk turns from left to right.

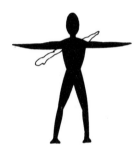

        Command: "And stop."
    3. Command: "Legs together."

C. *Arm exercise—front-support position (count of two, twenty times)*

Points to emphasize: Body should be straight. Correct breathing: inhale when bending, exhale when straightening. Strengthens arms, stomach and back.

    1. Command: "Down to front support at count two."
    2. Command: "Exercise at count two, begin."
        Count 1 Bend elbows, lowering body to ground.
        Count 2 Straighten elbows, raising body from ground.
        Command: "And stop."
    3. Command: "Upright position at count two."

D. *Trunk exercise—lying on back, hands clasped under chin (count of two, fifteen times)*

Points to emphasize: Back should round up. Strengthens stomach, chest and thighs.

1. Command: "Down to back at count two."
2. Command: "Exercise at count two, begin."

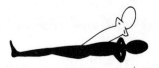

    Count 1 Lift upper part of trunk.
    Count 2 Lower upper part of trunk.
3. Command: "And stop."
4. Command: "Upright at count two."

STAGE IV: Drilling—32 Minutes

A. All points must be visible from instructor's position; equipment is set up in advance.
B. The instructor walks through the stations with the entire unit, explaining the designated exercise at each as one soldier demonstrates it twice.
C. Soldiers divide into ten groups, one group at each point. The instructor blows his whistle to signal the start of the exercise. Soldiers perform the designated exercise at each station as many times as possible until they hear the instructor's whistle (30 seconds). Then they run to the next station within 30 seconds and begin to exercise when the instructor whistles again.
D. An instructor or N.C.O. waits at each point to check on the correct performance of the exercise.
E. The chief instructor makes three successive rounds at all points.
F. Drill sequence:

    1. *Arm exercise—front-support position (count of two)*

    Points to emphasize: Keep body straight. Correct breathing: inhale when bending, exhale when straightening. Strengthens arms, back and stomach.

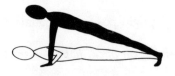

    Count 1 Bend elbows, lowering body to ground.
    Count 2 Straighten elbows, raising body from ground.

2. *Leg exercise—standing straight, facing bench or crate (60 cm. high) (count of four)*

   Points to emphasize: At counts two and four, legs are straight. Perform exercise at moderate rate. Strengthens thighs, calves and feet.

   > Count 1–2 Climb with right foot, followed by left; stand on bench.
   > Count 3–4 Climb down with right foot, followed by left; stand on ground.

3. *Back exercise—lying on stomach, facing wall; hands raised holding medicine ball*

   Points to emphasize: Perform exercise slowly. Aim for ball line on wall. Strengthens back, shoulders and arms.

   Tip: A line drawn on the wall 70 cm. from the ground will encourage soldiers to throw higher.

   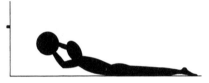

   Lie on stomach 1 meter from the wall. Throw a half-kilo medicine ball, aiming for the line. Catch it as it returns.

4. *Stomach exercise—lying on back, hands behind head, elbows out (count of two)*

   Points to emphasize: Keep back rounded throughout and legs straight.

   > Count 1 Rise to sitting position.
   > Count 2 Return to ground.

5. *Speed and quickness—lying on stomach*

   Points to emphasize: Front-support position precedes each sprint. Strengthens legs, increases agility and coordination.

   Spring up and sprint 10 meters. Sprint back to starting point and drop to front-support position.

6. *Arm exercise—suspension on ropes (count of two)*

   Points to emphasize: Keep legs off the ground. Strengthens arms and hands.

Count 1 Bend elbows, pulling body up until eyes are level with hands.

Count 2 Straighten elbows, lowering body.

7. *Jumping—legs slightly apart, 150 cm. from wall, medicine ball between feet.*

Points to emphasize: Aim consistently for the same height. Strengthens feet, calves, thighs and arms.

Pick up medicine ball with hands and throw toward wall while jumping. Aim between two lines on wall at heights of 80 and 120 cm. After each throw, trainee runs to retrieve ball and throws again.

8. *Stomach exercise—lying on back, legs straight with feet on bench (40 cm. high) 4 inches from wall, medicine ball between feet (count of two)*

Points to emphasize: Knees may be bent slightly. Develops stomach, thighs and feet.

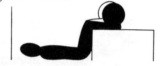

Count 1 Lift medicine ball to wall with straight legs about 6 inches.

Count 2 Lower medicine ball to bench with straight legs.

9. *Marksmanship*

Points to emphasize: Accuracy in hitting the pail. Throw medicine ball with both hands into pail on the ground 5 meters away. Run to pail at moderate pace to retrieve ball and return to starting position.

10. *Speed and quickness*

Points to emphasize: Develops legs and endurance and coordination.

Climb on and off a crate 40 cm. high as fast as possible.

STAGE V: Summation—5 Minutes

A. Unit is arranged in rows of threes.
B. Review of the lesson: Development of power, endurance, flexibility, agility and strength through a variety of exercises.
C. Questions and answers.

Lesson Plan #3

Subject of the lesson: Set exercise.

Goal: To develop physical ability.

Stages of the lesson and duration of each:

I.	Introduction	5 minutes
II.	400-meter run	3 minutes
III.	Warm-up calisthenics	5 minutes
IV.	Strength-building exercises	27 minutes
V.	Interval runs	5 minutes
VI.	Cool-down	5 minutes
	Total	50 minutes

SETTING UP THE LESSON

Location: The training area.

Instruction methods: Explanation, demonstration and drilling.

Training group: Unit of twenty to forty soldiers.

Preparation for instruction: Inspection of the training area.

Accessories and equipment: Parallel bars.

Clothing and gear: Military uniform, denim or gym clothes.

BREAKDOWN OF THE LESSON

STAGE I: Introducing the Lesson to the Unit—5 Minutes

A. The soldiers sit in rows.
B. *Opening*—The purpose of this lesson is to systematically develop physical ability through specific, very concentrated groups of strength-building exercises, called sets. Each set should be performed a minimum of three times a week, in the exact sequence they are presented here, at a rapid pace. The number of repeats should be increased by two each time the set is performed, thereby building strength and power and developing motivation through the constant setting and achievement of new goals.

STAGE II: The 400-Meter Run—3 Minutes

A. Arrange the unit in groups of three, facing in the direction they will run.
B. The soldiers sing or clap hands and run in rhythm at a moderate pace.
C. The instructor runs alongside and slightly behind the soldiers.
D. At the end of the run, the soldiers get into rows with their backs to the sun.

STAGE III: Warm-up Calisthenics—5 Minutes

Before each new exercise, the instructor demonstrates the complete movement, counting aloud and emphasizing specific points.

A. *Easy arm exercise—legs apart, hands behind head (count of four, eight times)*

   Points to emphasize: Pull stomach in.

   1. At the command "legs apart," soldiers jump into legs-apart position and place hands behind head, elbows out to sides.
   2. Command: "Exercise at count four, begin."

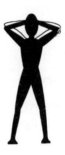

   Count 1–2 Pull arms back from the shoulder; bounce once.
   Count 3–4 Straighten arms to sides at shoulder height while pulling them back. Pull back again.
   3. Command: "And stop."
   4. Command: "Legs together."

B. *Trunk exercise—legs apart, arms extended upward (decreasing counts beginning with eight)*

   Points to emphasize: Bend trunk as much as possible.

   1. At the command "legs apart," soldiers jump into legs-apart position, and raise arms above head from shoulder.

2. Command: "Exercise begin."
>   Count 1–8 Bend trunk to the left and bounce seven times.
>   Count 1–8 Bend trunk to the right and bounce seven times.
>   Count 1–7 Bend trunk to the left and bounce six times.
>   Count 1–7 Bend trunk to the right and bounce six times.
>   Count 1–6 Bend trunk to the left and bounce five more times.
>   Count 1–6 Bend trunk to the right and bounce five more times.
>   Count 1–5 Bend trunk to the left and bounce four more times.
>   Count 1–5 Bend trunk to the right and bounce four more times.
>   Count 1–4 Bend trunk to the left and bounce three more times.
>   Count 1–4 Bend trunk to the right and bounce three more times.
>   Count 1–3 Bend trunk to the left and bounce twice more.
>   Count 1–3 Bend trunk to the right and bounce twice more.

3. Command: "Legs together, arms down."

C. *Trunk exercise—legs apart, trunk bent forward (count of two, fifteen times)*

Points to emphasize: Legs straight, increase pace.

1. At the command "legs apart," soldiers jump into legs-apart position and bend from the waist.
2. Command: "Exercise at count two, begin."
>   Count 1 Twist trunk to the left with a strong pull of both arms.

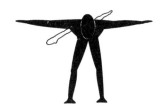

>   Count 2 Twist trunk to the right with a strong pull of both arms.
>   Command: "And stop."
>   At the command "legs together," soldiers straighten and jump into legs-together position.

D. *Trunk exercise—legs apart, arms extended upward (count of six, eight times)*

Points to emphasize: Straight legs.

1. Command: "Legs apart."
2. Command: "Exercise at count six, begin."

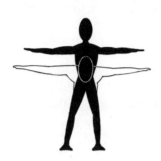

Count 1–4 Bend forward and bounce three times.
Count 5 Return to upright position, pulling arms up and back.
Count 6 Bounce arms back once.
3. Command: "And stop."
4. Command: "Legs together, arms down."

E. *Difficult arm exercise—very narrow front-support position (count of two, ten times)*

Points to emphasize: Keep legs straight. Correct breathing: inhale when bending, exhale when straightening.

1. Command: "Down to front support at count two."
2. Command: "Exercise at count two, begin."
   Count 1 Bend elbows, bringing chest as close as possible to hands.
   Count 2 Straighten elbows, raising body.
3. Command: "And stop."
4. Command: "Into upright position at count two."

STAGE IV: Strength-Building Exercises—27 Minutes

Before each exercise, the instructor slowly demonstrates the complete movement, counting aloud and emphasizing specific points. Exercises are performed in rounds of two, with a 30-second rest between rounds.

A. *Abdomen—lying on back, resting on forearms (count of two; two rounds of ten times each)*

Points to emphasize: Correct breathing: inhale while raising legs, exhale while lowering them.

   1. Command: "Down to back at count two."
   2. Command: "Exercise at count two, begin."
      Count 1 Slowly lift legs to a 90-degree angle.
      Count 2 Slowly lower legs to the ground.
   3. Command: "And rest." Soldiers rest for 30 seconds, then repeat exercise ten times at rhythm set by instructor, until command "and stop."
   4. Command: "Upright at count two."

B. *Arms and chest—front-support position (count of two; three rounds as indicated)*

Points to emphasize: Keep body and legs straight. Correct breathing: inhale while bending, exhale while straightening.

   1. Command: "Down to front support at count two."
   2. Command: "Exercise at count two, begin."

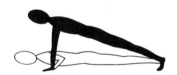

      Count 1 Bend elbows, bringing chest as close as possible to ground.
      Count 2 Straighten elbows, raising body.
     Perform exercise ten times.
   3. At the command "narrow front-support," soldiers decrease space between palms to 12 inches.
   4. Command: "Exercise at count two, begin."
      Count 1 Bend elbows, bringing chest as close as possible to ground.
      Count 2 Straighten elbows, raising body.
     Perform exercise six times.
   5. At the command "very narrow front support," soldiers move hands to palm-on-palm front-support position.
   6. Command: "Exercise at count two, begin."
      Count 1 Bend elbows, bringing chest as close to ground as possible.

      Count 2 Straighten elbows, raising body.
      Perform exercise two times.
  7. Command: "Upright at count two."

C. *Abdomen—lying on back, knees bent, legs held at ankles by partner (count of two; two rounds of twenty times to alternate sides)*

Points to emphasize: Correct breathing: exhale while rising, inhale while descending.

  1. Command: "Down to back at count two."
  2. Command: "Exercise at count two, begin."
      Count 1 Rise to sitting position, turning trunk to the left.
      Count 2 Return to starting position.
      Keep repeating to alternate sides as indicated above.
  3. Command: "Upright at count two."

D. *Arms and shoulders—suspension from parallel bar, broad overhand grip (count of two; two rounds of five times each)*

Points to emphasize: Correct breathing: exhale when pulling up, inhale when descending.

  1. Command: "Soldiers grasp bar."
  2. Command: "Exercise at count two, begin."
      Count 1 Bend elbows, raising body off ground until back of neck touches bar.
      Count 2 Straighten elbows, lowering body back to ground.

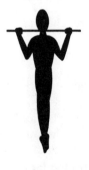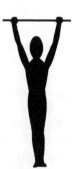

  3. Command: "And stop."

E. *Legs—partner on shoulders (count of two; two rounds of eight times each)*

Points to emphasize: Correct breathing: inhale when going down, exhale when rising. Heels to ground. Trunk straight.

1. Command: "Carry partner on shoulders." One soldier climbs on the shoulders of the other.
2. Command: "Exercise at count two, begin."
   Count 1 Bend knees to squatting position.
   Count 2 Straighten knees to upright position.
   Repeat two rounds of eight times each.
3. Command: "Change partners." Soldiers change positions, so that the carriers become the sitters. The new carriers perform two rounds of the exercise.
4. Command: "And stop."

STAGE V: Interval Runs—150 Meters, Eight Times—5 Minutes

A. Run in groups of five.
B. Time each group as it runs 150 meters as fast as they can.
C. Call out the times for each group. Each soldier checks his or her pulse. Pulse rate should not be above 190 beats per minute.
D. Run back to the starting point at a moderate pace (30 seconds for 150 meters). Each soldier checks his or her pulse rate again. Pulse rate should now be a maximum of 120 beats per minute.
E. Run the course at full speed eight times, return at a moderate pace eight times.

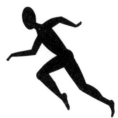

STAGE VI: Cool-down—5 Minutes

A. The entire unit runs 100 meters at a light pace.
B. Shift to rhythmic walking.

Lesson Plan #4

Subject of the lesson: Nature trip.

Goal: To develop physical ability while moving through an open area.

Stages of the lesson and duration of each:

I.	Introduction	5 minutes
II.	400-meter run	3 minutes
III.	Calisthenics	6 minutes
IV.	Games and strength-building in an open area	30 minutes
V.	Cool-down and summation	6 minutes
	Total	50 minutes

SETTING UP THE LESSON

Location: Sandy, hilly area.

Instruction methods: Explanation, demonstration and drilling.

Training group: A unit of twenty to forty soldiers.

Preparation for instruction: Inspection of training area and route.

Training accessories and equipment: Two canteens, one whistle, beam, stones, barrel.

Clothing and gear: Military uniform or gym clothes; army shoes or sneakers.

BREAKDOWN OF THE LESSON

STAGE I: Introducing the Lesson to the Unit—5 Minutes

This lesson is designed to develop physical ability and awareness of one's surroundings, to use the terrain to one's best advantage in field exercises, maneuvers and combat situations. A diversity of outdoor areas can be used. Imagination and motivation are much more important in this lesson than the others.

STAGE II: The 400-Meter Run—3 Minutes

A. The unit is arranged in threes. Roll call. Make sure canteens are full.
B. Instructor runs in front. Running need not be in threes.

STAGE III: Calisthenics—6 Minutes

A. *Easy arm exercise*
Forward and backward circular movements with arms while walking for 50 meters.

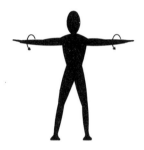

B. *Trunk exercise with 30-meter forward movement (count of four)*
Count 1–2 Two steps forward and two arm pulls upward and backward.
Count 3–4 With legs apart and arms outstretched, bend and bounce once.

C. *50-meter walk*
Take large steps foward and loosely swing arms toward the side of the leg that is in front, turning trunk slightly.

D. *Front-facing trunk exercise—legs apart and arms lifted (count of two, twenty times)*
Count 1–2 Bend trunk from side to side.

STAGE IV: Games and Strength-Building in Open Area—30 Minutes

A. *Walking on all fours and "hideaway" (two times over a 40-meter range)*

1. The soldiers advance on all fours.
2. On hearing the whistle, each runs into hiding within 20 seconds.
3. Those who can be spotted from the instructor's position must return on all fours.

B. *Forward hopping*

    1. Unit divides into groups of four.
    2. The first in each group stands in "leapfrog" position.
    3. The second in line leaps over him and stands 2 meters beyond him.
    4. The game continues over a distance of 30 meters.

C. *Equilibrium*
Cross a trench on a beam, pipe, log, etc.

D. *Barrel hitting*

    1. The soldiers pair off. Each soldier has three stones.
    2. Marksmanship competition: Each pair in turn throws its stones. The pair making the most noise by hitting the barrel wins, based on the instructor's decision.

E. *Abdominal exercises—lying on back, hands behind head (count of two; twenty times in free rhythm)*

    Count 1 Rise to sitting position.
    Count 2 Return to starting position.

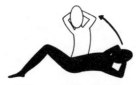

F. *Attack and defense—"King of the Hill"*

    1. All climb the hill.
    2. At a signal given by the instructor, all try to push the others off the hill.
    3. The last to remain on the hill is the winner.

G. *Endurance*

    1. Soldiers pair off.
    2. One soldier carries a friend on his shoulders, over a 200-meter distance.
    3. Each carrier becomes the passenger, and carrier walks back the 200-meter distance.

STAGE V: Cool-down and Summation—6 Minutes

A. Unit arranges itself in threes.
B. Walk to the base.
C. Sound a cheer!

Individualized Programs for Men and Women

THE I.D.F. COMBAT FITNESS DIVISION has developed an individualized program that does away with those standard excuses about lack of time, lack of equipment, lack of money or lack of guidance. The 20-minute methods for men and women provide the exact direction that those who prefer to work on their own need for a well-rounded, effective fitness program.

Simply use either method three times a week and you will soon see improvement. The exercises are extremely simple, require no special facilities, and can be adjusted to a specific fitness level and rate of progress. It can, of course, be adapted for groups.

The 20-Minute Method for Men

WARM-UP—2 MINUTES

1. Stand straight: Jump up, spreading legs apart, and swing arms out and above head; then jump up, closing legs and swing arms down to starting position—1 minute.

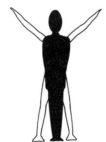

2. Legs apart: Bend forward, touch toes. Return to initial position—1 minute.

Exercise—1–5 Minutes Total

	Poor	Fair	Good	Very Good
1. Sit-ups				
18 to 26 years old:	15	30	50	60
26 to 36 years old:	10	15	30	50
36 and over:	8	10	15	30
2. Push-ups				
18 to 26 years old:	12	20	30	40
26 to 36 years old:	8	12	20	30
36 and over:	5	8	12	20
3. Lie on stomach, forehead to ground, hands extended forward. Clap in front and behind back.				
18 to 26 years old:	30	40	50	60
27 to 36 years old:	20	30	40	50
37 and over:	10	20	30	40
4. Squat-thrust				
18 to 26 years old:	10	20	25	30
27 to 36 years old:	6	10	20	25
37 and over:	4	6	10	20
5. Sprints (40 meters × 3)— running at full speed				
18 to 26 years old:	8 sec.	7	6.5	6
27 to 36 years old:	10	8	7	6.5
37 and over:	12	10	8	7

Endurance—2,500 Meters

Long-distance running	Poor	Fair	Good	Very Good
18 to 26 years old:	16:30–14:30	14:29–12:01	12:00–10:16	10:15 and under
26 to 36 years old:	17:30–15:30	15:29–13:01	13:00–11:16	11:15 and under
36 and over:	18:30–16:30	16:29–14:01	14:00–12:16	12:15 and under

COOL-DOWN—1 MINUTE

Bend forward at the waist, then straighten while raising arms (knees slightly bent, legs apart)

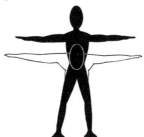

Exhale when bending, inhale when rising. Do it slowly and easily.
Total—20 Minutes

GUIDELINES FOR TRAINING

1. Find a suitable place with plenty of room and a cushioned surface (grass or sand outdoors, a carpeted floor indoors) for training. You'll lessen the chance of injury.
2. Ability should determine the number of exercises you do or how far you run. Don't strain yourself.
3. Do not sit down immediately after exercising or running. Walk to cool down.
4. Keep track of your progress and keep trying to improve.
5. Work toward your desired score gradually and persistently until you succeed in attaining it.

The 20-Minute Method for Women

WARM-UP—2 MINUTES

1. Stand straight: Jump up, spreading legs apart, and raising arms above head; then jump again, closing legs and returning arms to the sides. Repeat for 1 minute.

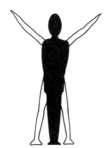

2. Legs apart and hands on waist: Perform trunk turns to the right and to the left for 1 minute.

STRENGTH AND POWER—3 MINUTES

Exercise up to 1 minute each	Poor	Fair	Good	Very Good
1. Sit-ups:				
16 to 24 years old:	8–19	20–29	30–34	45 and over
25 to 30 years old:	6–17	18–24	25–39	40 and over
31 and over:	5–14	15–21	22–34	35 and over
2. Six-point push-ups:				
16 to 24 years old:	5–9	10–14	15–24	25 and over
25 to 30 years old:	4–7	8–11	12–21	22 and over
31 and over:	3–5	6–9	10–19	20 and over
3. Lie on stomach, forehead on ground, hands extended forward. Clap hands in front and behind back.				
16 to 24 years old:	15–19	20–29	30–39	40 and over
25 to 30 years old:	12–15	16–24	25–31	32 and over
31 and over:	10–13	14–21	22–27	28 and over

ENDURANCE—1,500 METERS

Long-distance running	Poor	Fair	Good	Very Good
16 to 24 years old:	12:00–10:01	10:00–8:01	8:00–6:51	6:50 or under
25 to 30 years old:	14:00–12:01	12:00–10:01	10:00–8:51	8:50 or under
31 and over:	16:00–14:01	14:00–12:01	12:00–10:51	10:50 or under

COOL-DOWN—5 MINUTES

1. Shift to walking for 2 minutes.
2. Walk while "throwing legs" for 2 minutes.
3. Light forward trunk bends while exhaling. Straighten up and pull arms upward while inhaling (knees slightly bent, feet apart) for 1 minute.

Total—20 Minutes

GUIDELINES FOR TRAINING

1. Find a place with plenty of room and a cushioned surface (grass or sand outdoors, a carpeted floor indoors) for training. You'll lessen the chance of injury.
2. Ability should determine the number of exercises you do or how far you run. Don't strain yourself.
3. Do not sit down immediately after exercising or running. Walk to cool down.
4. Keep track of your progress and keep trying to improve.
5. Work toward your desired score gradually and persistently until you succeed in attaining it.

WORK OUT EVERY DAY AND YOU'RE SURE TO SUCCEED!

Fitness for Youth Prior to Recruitment

The Combat Fitness Department is keenly interested in the physical fitness of young people about to be recruited into the I.D.F. The young men and women should reach a minimal level of fitness in order to meet the demands of the initial training period. Every young person should be concerned about his or her own physical fitness and should develop a set of activities and goals for self-improvement. Increased challenges will motivate young people to do their best and to improve upon their previous achievements. In Israel, the I.D.F. has developed a challenging fitness program that is in use in high schools throughout the country.

Youth around the world have come to understand that life in modern society can be healthier and more beneficial by staying in shape. Let us present our young people with the kind of simple tasks they will have to perform when they enter the army. We've tried to be realistic in order not to create frustration among the young people taking part in the exercises and tests. We are not dealing with outstanding athletes. Our target population consists of a majority of 17- to 19-year-olds, who should be in good physical condition.

Rise and Shine

WHAT DO YOU DO when you start the day? Do you get off to a brisk start and make the most of whatever you do? These exercises show the great variety of ways to develop fitness as part of everyday activities. But they are only some examples. You can easily make up your own.

At a leisurely pace, they will increase your circulation, improve your disposition, and bolster your vitality. Performed at a rigorous pace, they will improve your physical condition.

Don't walk to the shower. *Run* at an even pace.

After washing your face, place your hands on the sink for some knee-bends. Get all the way down without letting go, then rise slowly to standing position.

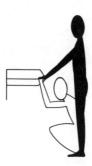

Keep your hands on the sink and move your legs straight back, feet flat on the floor. Bend your elbows as far as you can, then straighten them again. Do not bend your knees.

Even if the kitchen is very near, make a point of running. While waiting for the kettle to boil, keep running in place, lifting your knees as high as you can. Next, try kicking your heels as close to your buttocks as you can.

Don't lift your foot onto a stool to tie your shoes. Instead, get down to squatting position.

Now that your shoes are on, stand with legs apart and slowly bend your body forward from the waist, stretching your arms out in front of you. The return should be gradual, not sudden. Repeat several times.

Fitness for the Office Worker

JUST LIKE CIVILIANS, many soldiers spend most of their time sitting in an office—and getting out of shape. It's for such chair-bound office workers that we'd like to suggest some suitable exercises. Most of these are isometric, which means that they involve activating a muscle against an object whose force is equal to or greater than that of the muscle. The exercise itself does not involve any movement; i.e., the effort is static.

If you faithfully do these exercises every day, you'll increase your strength and firm your muscles, but will do little to improve your endurance and flexibility. This program is not as effective as the 20-minute methods, but for some it has its advantages. It's perfect for truly dedicated office workers.

1. Stand facing the wall at a distance of about 20 inches, with your body inclined forward, hands on the wall. Run in place for 1 minute. Pause and repeat.

2. Stand in the doorframe, hands to the sides and push for 7 seconds. Release. Do it ten times.

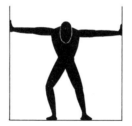

3. Sit on a chair, press hands together, elbows at 90-degree angles, for 7 seconds. Release. Do it ten times.

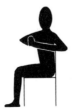

4. Stay seated. Raise your legs until they are parallel to the floor. Place your feet against a wall and push for 7 seconds. Release. Push ten times.

5. Still seated, hold your arms out with elbows bended at 90-degree angles. Grasp left wrist with right hand. Now try to break that grasp by pulling your elbows in opposite directions. After a few pulls, switch grasp to other hand and repeat.

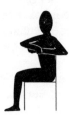

6. Sitting on your chair, push down on the floor while at the same time pushing your back against the back of the chair. Hold for 7 seconds. Release. Do it ten times.

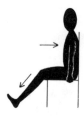

7. Stand away from the desk, legs together, hands flat on the desk. Rise on your toes, then bend your knees, lowering yourself into squatting position, arms extended forward. Return to standing position. Repeat several times.

8. Stand with your side to the desk. Place the leg nearest the desk on the desk, unbended. Bend twice toward the raised leg, twice to the center and twice to the standing leg. Repeat several times. Switch legs and continue.

9. Stand facing the chair (be sure it's sturdy and has straight legs). Step on to the seat, as though climbing a stair. Step back down. Repeat twenty times.

10. Stand with your back to the chair. Take hold of the seat and bring your body into reverse-support position. Bend elbows and lower yourself toward the floor, keeping your body straight, then return to starting position. Repeat ten times.

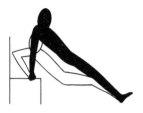

11. Stand with legs apart, hands on hips. Alternately bend twice to the right, then twice to the left. Rest for two counts in center. Repeat several times.

Let Your Home Furniture Help You to Better Health and Fitness

WHEN NOT ON ACTIVE DUTY, the Israeli soldier keeps fit at home. Furniture can be used for exercising and getting or staying in shape. Exercising at home with the whole family is not only good for your health but can be a great source of fun and recreation. Here are some exercises that use common household furniture and encourage spouses or roommates to join you. These are suggestions. Think of some on your own.

A. A Chair—*Abdomen*

Lying on your back, with your legs on the chair and hands behind your head, rise to sitting position. If this proves too difficult, rise only to the point where shoulders and chest are off the ground. Repeat five to twenty times.

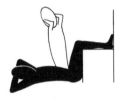

B. A Carpet—*Arm Muscles*

In six-point position, bend your elbows, lowering trunk until chin touches the ground. After practicing, try doing the same exercise from front-support position. Repeat ten to forty times.

C. A Broom—*Shoulders*

Hold the broom above your head, with arms apart. Pull arms back as far as possible without bending elbows and return to starting position. Repeat ten to forty times.

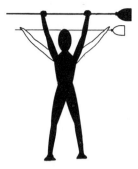

D. A Table—*Back*

Lying facedown on a table or bed, move forward until your entire trunk is hanging over the edge. Have someone hold your legs so that you don't lose your balance. Putting your arms behind your head, arch your body so that trunk is higher than the tabletop. Return to starting position.

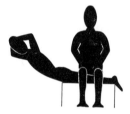

E. Books (or Other Heavy Objects)—*Legs*

Lying on your back, place two books (or only one at first) across both ankles. With legs together, lift as slowly as possible from the floor to a 30-degree angle, then return to starting position.

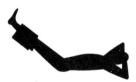

F. Exercising in Pairs—*Endurance*

Stand facing one another. One partner demonstrates different ways of jumping as the other imitates him. Change roles after 1 minute. Suggestions: jump on one leg, or feet apart, or stepping forward and back, etc.

Advice and Exercises for Your Back

THE PREREQUISITES FOR preventing back pains are:
1. Reinforce abdominal and back muscles.
2. Increase the flexibility of your spine.
3. Be aware of how your spine works and of its position during the course of the day. Take care of your back.

Back pains interfere with many people's ability to work and enjoy life. There are numerous causes of back pains, from incorrect sitting posture or toting an overstuffed briefcase to the simple accumulation of years of bearing down on the spine.

One way of preventing back pains or at least minimizing them is to reinforce the lumbar region by strengthening the back and abdominal muscles.

Begin by standing straight and stretching your spinal column upward. Repeat this several times in the course of the day until it becomes a habit. Next, do exercises described below. We recommend that you do these every day.

1. *Warm-up—Tensing and relaxing (ten to thirty times)*

   Lie on back with knees bent. Exhale as you bring the left knee to the chest. Inhale as you return to starting position. Alternate knees.

2. *Back exercise (ten to thirty times)*

   Lie on stomach with arms at sides. Inhale. Exhale while lifting arms, and breathe freely. Don't raise your limbs too high, or perform this exercise too quickly. Inhale as you return to starting position.

3. *Abdominal exercise (ten to fifty times)*

   Inhale while lying on back, hands behind head. Exhale while raising trunk off the floor to a 45-degree angle. Stay in this position, breathing freely, for several seconds before returning to floor.

4. *Loosening exercise (ten to twenty times each side)*

   Lie on back with knees bent to chest. Move knees to the right and to the left while exhaling, in a slow horizontal motion. Inhale when knees touch floor.

Posture Tips

A. *Sitting posture for drivers of armored vehicles (or any vehicle)*

Drivers will have their share of back pains unless they heed the rules of correct posture. There should be some form of support, such as a cushion, for the lumbar region when sitting in an armored combat vehicle or most vehicles. The seat must also be comfortable, since the vertical and horizontal movements of the seat can jolt the spinal column, causing irritation and back pains.

B. *How to lift a shell (or other heavy object)*

In the army, the artillerist's main problem comes from lifting shells of varying weight. Incorrect lifting puts a tremendous strain on the back and can damage the lumbar region of the spinal column. The soldier, or any individual, should learn how to lift heavy objects correctly and build up those muscle systems that take part in the lifting operation.

The illustration below shows a soldier trying to lift a heavy shell at an incorrect angle, using his back muscles. Severe harm to the muscles and vertebrae is likely to result.

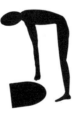

The correct approach, illustrated below, is to bring the shell or heavy object as close to the body as possible and, bending the legs to a squatting position, use the leg muscles for lifting. The leg muscles relieve much of the burden from the back.

A tray may also be used for lifting shells. Here, too, the brunt is on the leg muscles, to ease the load on the back.

PART II

Self-Defense—
Contact Combat

The Need for Self-Defense

YOU'RE WALKING ALONG, stopping now and again to look into shop windows, glancing at movie theaters with their pictures of violence from the latest films. You buy the evening paper and read about assault, rape, murder, and other hair-raising news as you go from headline to headline. You walk on and treat yourself to an ice-cream cone to make your own pleasant life even sweeter. Yours is a peaceful existence. It goes on this way for years. All around you, you hear about violence, read about violence, and see violence on television and in movies, but in your heart of hearts, you think (or hope) that it could never happen to you—because it never has. The maelstrom of violence simply threatens to engulf you, as far as you're concerned it's as far away as ever.

But on one of those evenings, a group of rowdy youths closes in on you without warning. A heavy blow to your legs leaves you stretched out on the pavement. The loud laughter of your assailants accompanies a sharp kick in your ribs. You struggle to your feet, start to run, and get boxed in the face. You feel a kick in the stomach. Your hands flail. You stagger about and do your best to get as far away as possible. The path finally becomes clear when the gang has had its share of fun and has lost interest in you.

It can happen to anyone—a situation of utter helplessness, panic and fear. You showed no ingenuity, no orientation or inclination to use your empty hands for your own defense. Your sense of confidence evaporated with the first blow. The only way to restore it is to learn self-defense techniques, in case you are ever again in a similar situation.

Self-Defense in the World

DAY IN AND DAY OUT we hear about karate, judo, jujitsu, aikido, boxing, wrestling and other methods of defending oneself with or without side arms. The experts all go to great lengths to explain the merits of each system, touting not only its effectiveness in warding off an assailant, but also its dignity, its inner discipline, its ability to improve powers of concentration, its focus on important educational values and consideration for others, and its capability to instill self-confidence, agility, speedy reflexes, the capacity to withstand blows and the ability to respond in kind.

It soon becomes obvious, however, that these arts of combat are a complete way of life. Martial arts training requires a high degree of specialization and consistent adherence to the particular tradition and approach of each school. A man must devote years of his life before he can hope to reach the level of skill and mastery that would render him capable of putting his knowledge to use for his own defense.

The Israel Defense Forces System of Self-Defense

THE I.D.F. NEEDED a system that would work quickly for anyone and everyone. Over the past thirty years, we developed the Contact Combat Program. Among its unique features are:

Simplicity—The exercises are easy to learn, easy to perform, uncomplicated and straightforward.

Short-term instruction—The idea is to teach the system within three weeks of intensive training.

Clarity and purposefulness—There are a definite number of exercises, each with a definite goal.

Use of side arms—Weapons are used as tools. Soldiers are taught rapid reactions in case a weapon is jammed or empty.

Adaptability—Correct response is taught in a trench, a bunker, a field, a courtyard, a street—*anywhere.*

Techniques—Basic elements have been taken from other arts of self-defense, adapted to I.D.F. needs.

Proficiency—The only standard to be attained is the actual performance of the exercise and its immediate effect.

One Program for All

WHAT MUST YOU, an average person, make sure to learn in anticipation of self-defense situations in today's violent world? You must know your own body well: your movements, reactions, speed, orientation and the way you behave under pressure or in unfamiliar situations. You must be able to receive blows, feel pain, and learn how to overcome them and to avoid panic. This means receiving one blow after another, falling down, having your hair pulled, and knowing how to look, to think, and to keep your cool through it all. Your next challenge is to learn to use your own arms and legs as effectively as possible against your assailant.

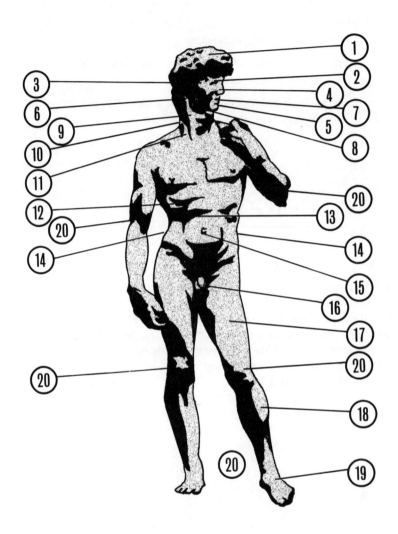

Vulnerable Points of the Human Body

A. *To deliver an effective blow, you must be familiar with the vulnerable points in the body:*

1. Hair (for gripping)
2. Eyes
3. Temples
4. Nose (nasal bridge and top of nose)
5. Chin
6. Ear
7. Mouth
8. Throat
9. Sides of the neck
10. Back of the neck
11. Clavicle hollow and throat
12. Ribs
13. Kidneys
14. Waist and hips
15. Stomach
16. Testicles
17. Thigh
18. Calf and shin
19. Top of foot
20. All joints and articulations: shoulders, elbows, wrists, fingers, knees, ankles, toes, spine.

B. *Actions that cause injury:*

1. Kicking
2. Hitting
3. Pressure and strangulation
4. Pulling and biting
5. Leverage against a joint

C. *Types of injury:*

1. trauma, severe pain (broken bone, kick in the groin)
2. knockout (punch in the chin)
3. death (broken neck)

D. *Manner of injuring vulnerable points:*
  1. *Hair*—Hand slides into hair with fingers apart, near scalp. The fingers are clamped shut and the hand pulls from left to right and down. The hair is regarded more as a grabbing point than a vulnerable point per se.
  2. *Eyes*—Thumb pressure or jabbing with index finger (severe trauma).
  3. *Temples*—Fist punch with the second joint of the middle finger protruding or finger jab.
  4. *Nose*—Fist punch, hammer blow (on the nasal bridge); fifth-finger or karate-type blow to base of nose; or pressure on top of nose (stunning).
  5. *Chin*—Fist punch, karate-type chop, elbow blow, hand blow (stunning).
  6. *Ears*—Tearing, biting, punching (stunning).
  7. *Mouth*—Fist punch, karate-type chop, elbow blow, tearing (stunning).
  8. *Throat*—Karate-type chop, fist punch, strangulation (stunning, death).
  9. *Neck*—Karate-type blow (severe trauma); strangulation (death).
  10. *Back of neck*—Karate-type blow, hammer blow (death).
  11. *Clavicle hollow*—Severe pressure, stabbing with knife (death).
  12. *Ribs*—Fist punch, karate-type chop, elbow blow, kicking, stomping (stunning).
  13. *Kidneys*—Karate-type blow, fist punch, kicking (severe trauma).
  14. *Waist and hips*—Karate-type chop, kicks (severe trauma).
  15. *Stomach*—Kicking, fist punch (severe trauma).
  16. *Testicles*—Kicking, hitting (severe trauma); pressure (death).
  17. *Thighs*—Kicking (severe trauma).
  18. *Shins*—Kicking (severe trauma).
  19. *Top of foot*—Stomping (severe trauma).
  20. *All joints and articulations:* Fracture or dislocation by applying leverage against the direction of movement or in the direction of movement with a kick or blow.
      Knees—Kick, elbow blow (severe trauma).
      Ankles—Kick, elbow blow (severe trauma).
      Shoulders—Fist punch, two-handed grip (severe trauma).
      Elbows—Two-handed grip (severe trauma).
      Wrists—One- or two-handed grip (severe trauma).
      Fingers—Grip and bend (severe trauma).
      Spine—Kick and blow (severe trauma).
      Toes—Blow with the heel (severe trauma).

Learning the Contact Combat Program

THE SOLDIERS OF the I.D.F. train to be good contact combatants within three weeks. Their course is very demanding—seven to ten hours a day under the direction of a highly qualified instructor. If you practice for at least 15 minutes three times a week, you'll soon see results.

Begin by learning the basics—starting position, falling, blows and kicks. At first, concentrate on perfecting the movement itself. Then work on accuracy. Pick a spot or an object, and try to come as close as possible to striking it with a blow or kick. Once you begin to consistently hit your mark, work on speed. Your movements will be most effective if you are fast *and* accurate. Do five exercises each time you practice.

Once your basic movements are proficient, begin work with a partner. If your practice sessions have been less than an hour, you may want to extend them.

Work with a partner is important to improve reflexes and reactions. Begin by practicing the combinations of movements in this book. When you have learned them, make up ones of your own. Each should try to outwit the other. Remember—the more you practice, the better you'll become.

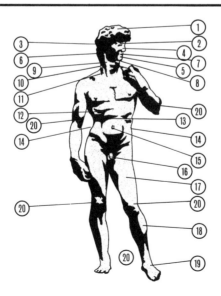

Basic Positions and Movements

THE BASIC POSITIONS and movements are standing, moving, rolling and blocking. They are essential to effective fighting in both offense and defense. In battle, basic positions and movements are not final. They are used to gain a more advantageous position against the opponent. The battle goes on and the fighter must continue to attack and to defend him or herself. Remember, your first priority in any combat situation is to protect yourself and to avoid being struck.

Points to emphasize:

1. Try to perfect the movement itself first. Have a friend check your stability in the standing position by pushing you from the front or from behind. If you lose your balance, adjust your stance until you can hold your ground.

2. Once you have perfected the standing position, add movement. Take a step to the left, to the right, and forward and backward. Be sure to move both feet, not simply widen your stance.

3. Work on speed and accuracy.

4. The instructions are given for one side, but they can easily be adapted to the other by substitution, e.g., left for right. Practice *both* sides.

EXERCISE 1 STARTING POSITION

1. Begin with legs about 14 inches apart.

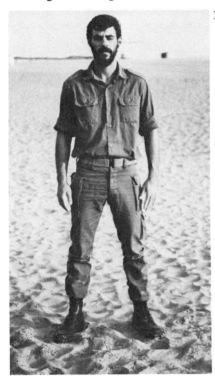

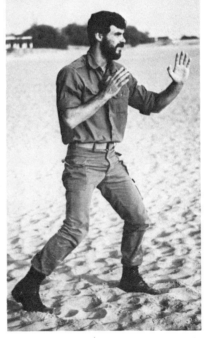

2. Advance left foot about 14 inches, turning foot slightly inward. Raise right heel and look up. Weight is on both feet, with 60 percent of the weight on the front (left) foot. Body is turned about 65 degrees. Bend arms up at elbows. Hands should be at shoulder height: the right hand extended 12 inches from the body and the left extended 18 inches from the body. Hands should be angled out.

EXERCISE 2 180-DEGREE DEFENSE AGAINST BLOWS AND KICKS

Points to emphasize:

1. Practice each defense until movement is correct. Then combine them into a smooth arc from overhead to ground.
2. Use the back of forearm when blocking. The movement will be stronger and more natural, and the chance of injury reduced.
3. Make sure your hand is stiff.

Starting position—Legs slightly apart, one leg slightly forward, arms at sides.

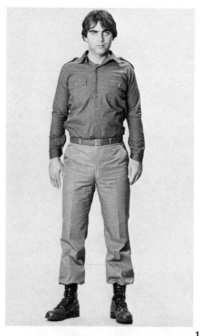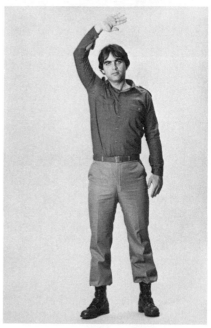

1

Defense #1—Raise right hand and forearm above head, palm out. There should be a 120-degree angle between upper arm and forearm, with the upper arm close to right ear.

Defense #2—Hand and arm move down 45 degrees. Palm faces out. Angle between arm and forearm decreases to 90 degrees.

Defense #3—Move arm down until upper arm is straight out from shoulder, forearm straight up, so that angle between upper arm and forearm is 90 degrees. Palm forward.

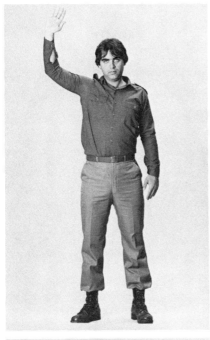

2

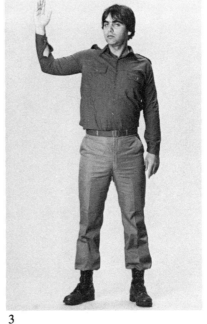

3

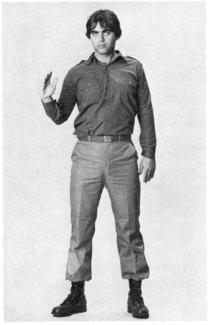

4

Defense #4—Bring upper arm down 45 degrees, so that elbow aligns with right toe. Maintain a 45-degree angle between upper arm and forearm, palm forward.

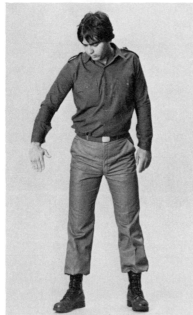

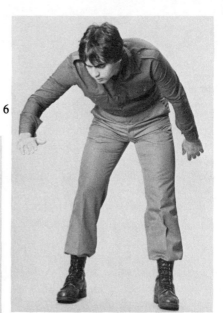

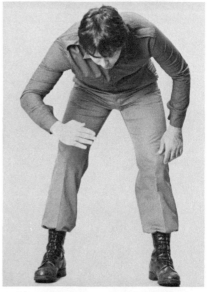

Defense #5—Draw forearm down, so that it is vertical to ground, palm facing back.

Defense #6—Bend trunk forward and to the right, most of weight rests on right foot. There should be a 120-degree angle between upper arm and forearm, so that forearm aligns with face.

Defense #7—Bend body forward, body weight rests evenly on both feet. Upper arm is perpendicular to ground; maintain a 120-degree angle between arm and forearm, palm turned in.

Exercise 3 Backward Blocking

1. Starting position—Stand straight, with legs slightly apart.
2. Sit close to heels without touching the ground. Arms crossed at wrists (right over left if you are right-handed) in front of chest.
3. Keeping rear close to left leg, roll backward until shoulders hit the ground. Raise arms frely. Do not raise pelvis off the ground.

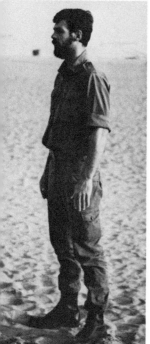

1

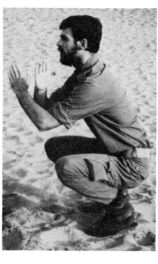

2

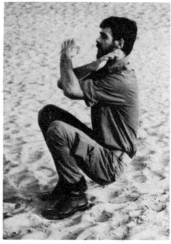

3

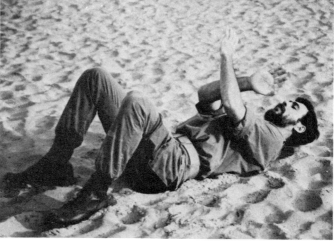

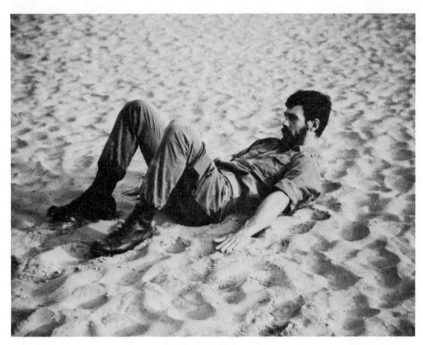

4. Drop hands to sides, 8 inches from body, fingers together. Press down on hand and forearm, raise head and shoulders.

5. Raise right foot, bent at ankle, ready for heel kick.

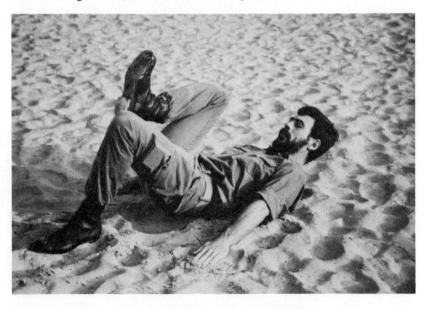

EXERCISE 4 BLOCKING SIDEWAYS

1. Starting position—Legs slightly apart.
2. Swing arms to the left, right arm to shoulder height, back of hand toward face. Draw right leg to the left in front of left leg.

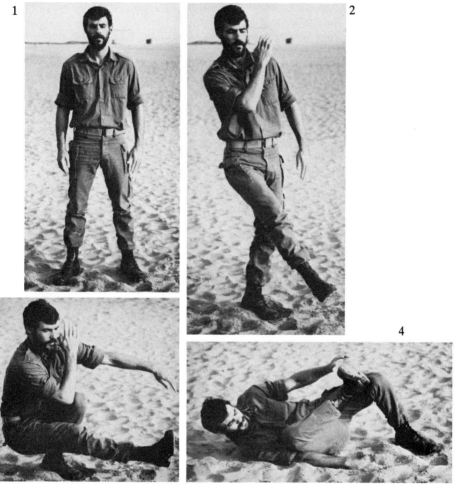

3. Squat on left leg, keeping right leg raised.
4. Lie on right side, left leg bent, head bent toward stomach, upper body curled slightly. Right arm is beside and slightly away from body. Right hand and forearm break the fall. Left hand is in front of chest, close to body. Right leg is bent in preparation for kick. Practice falling so that arm, from hand to elbow, consistently hits the ground at the same time.

EXERCISE 5 FRONT ROLL (SOMERSAULT) OVER RIGHT SHOULDER

1. Starting position—Legs slightly apart.
2. Step forward with right leg. Bend forward and place hands on ground, about 4 inches apart and turned in. Most of weight is on right hand.
3. Bend arms and roll over right shoulder, landing on left side of pelvis. Left leg is bent, shin under right knee.
4. Continue to roll forward and rise on left knee. Right foot is 10 inches away, and in line with knee. Rest on the balls of the feet.
5. Stand up. Turn to the left, about 45 degrees, stand on balls of feet. Assume the starting position (Exercise 1).

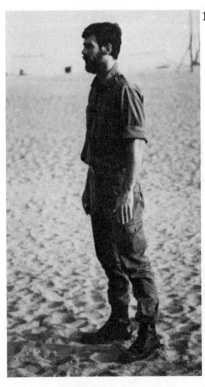

1

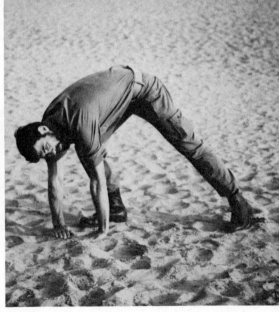

2

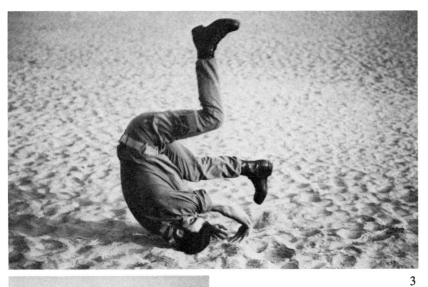

3

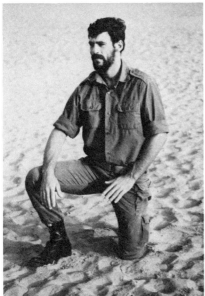

4

5

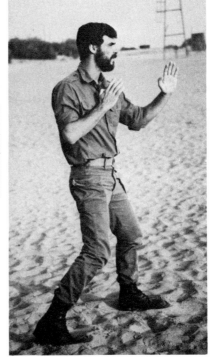

Exercise 6 Back Roll

1. Starting position—Legs slightly apart.
2. Right leg shifts back about 20 inches, toes in line with left foot.
3. Bend right knee until shin touches ground, trunk inclined slightly forward, arms to the left.
4. Roll backward, left knee over left shoulder and right leg straight back.
5. Land on balls of feet. Use hands to get up. Resume starting position (Exercise 1).

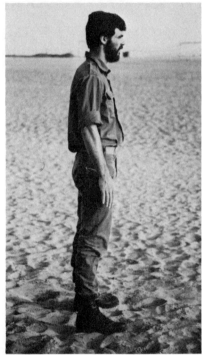

1

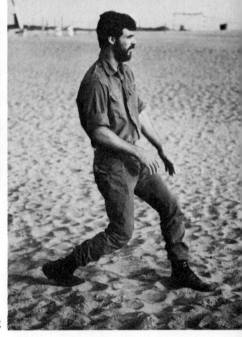

2

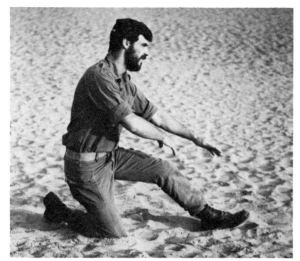

3

4

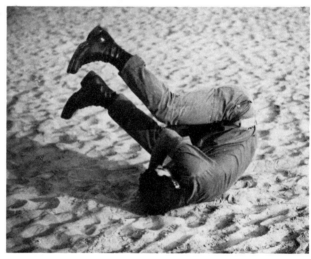

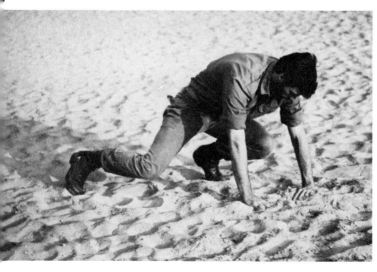

Blows

TEACHING THE ART OF hitting and punching ensures the effective use of the hands as weapons. The principles of an effective blow are:

A. Shaping the hand most effectively to cause injury—fist, palm, side of hand, etc.
B. Concentration.
C. Using body weight, strength and speed to the best advantage.
D. Accurate aim at the correct point.

Points to emphasize:

1. Steps are shown for a blow with the right hand. For left-hand blows, simply substitute right for left in the instructions. Practice with both left and right hands.
2. Begin practice while standing in place. Concentrate on performing the movement correctly, then on accuracy and speed.
3. When you've achieved accuracy and speed, do the exercise while moving forward, backward, and to either side.
4. Exercise 1 is the basic starting position for each exercise in this section unless otherwise indicated.
5. Some of the exercises are shown with a partner, but when you begin, practice by yourself until you achieve speed and accuracy.

EXERCISE 7 CLENCHING FIST

1. Fingers straight, close together. Thumb away from fingers.
2. Curl fingers at second knuckle.
3. Curl fingers at large knuckle.
4. Close fist very tightly, with thumb between second and third finger.

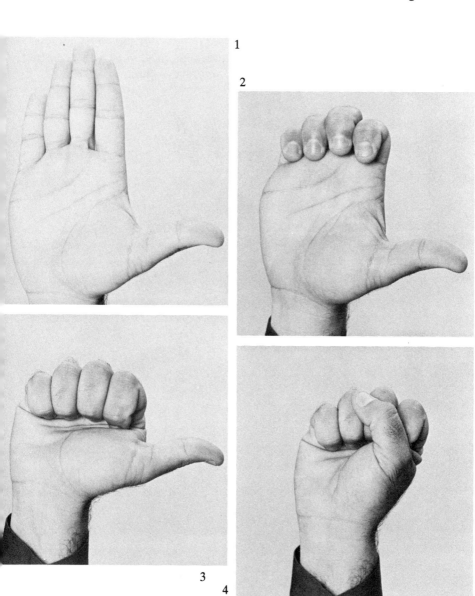

EXERCISE 8 FIST BLOW

1. Starting position.
2. As right arm is straightened, curl hand into a fist, fingers pointed down, and turn trunk to the left. Flex arm muscles. Elbow is down and bent slightly. DO NOT lock elbow. Push weight into punch with left leg. Left elbow back, forearm near body, fingers at chin height.
3. Fist hits target at the two blackened points. Fist should be horizontal. Aim for the center of the attacker's face when you begin to practice. As accuracy improves, aim for his chin.

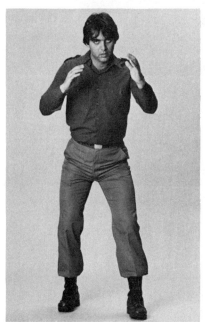

1

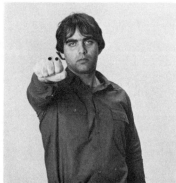

2

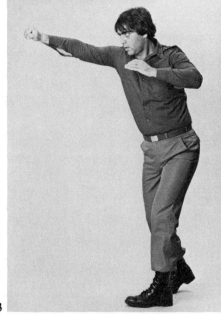

3

EXERCISE 9 PUNCH TO THE STOMACH

1. Starting position.
2. Advance with left foot one step, so that foot is at center of body, weight on left leg. Bend knees, lean trunk forward. Extend right arm in direct blow to attacker's stomach. Right arm should be bent at elbow so that palm is in front and slightly to the left of your face for protection.

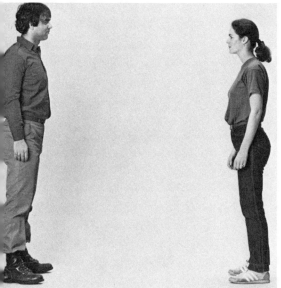

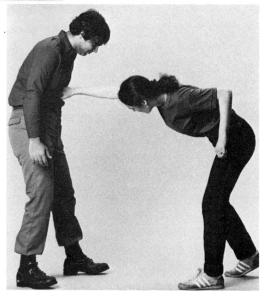

EXERCISE 10 HAMMER BLOW

1. Starting position.
2. Lift right hand, clenching fist at head height.
3. Bring hand straight down. Bend knees slightly. Hand is vertical; outer edge strikes blow. This blow is most effective if the attacker is bent over.

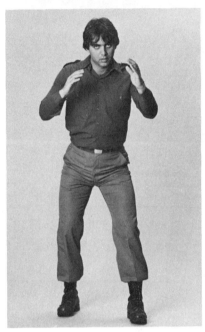

1

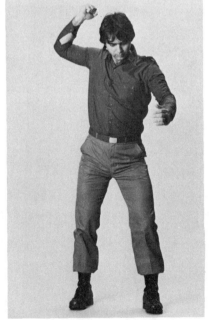

2

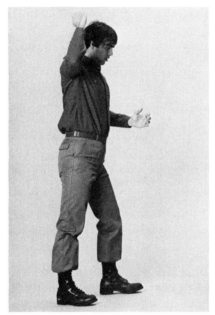

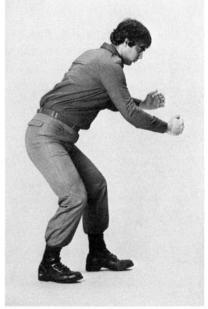

3

Exercise 11 Blows with Fingers and Knuckles

1. *Protruding knuckle punch*—Clench fist, but keep large knuckle of middle finger straight, thumb closed over it, so that middle knuckle of middle finger protrudes. Execute punch the same as closed fist (see Exercise 8). This blow is more accurate than a straight fist, but it's not as strong. Use this blow to the temple to kill, or to the diaphragm, to the throat, or to the groin for a more severe injury than a straight fist would inflict.

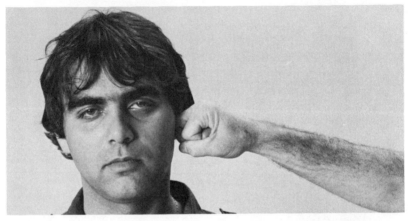

2. *Finger jab*—Fingers are close together and straight. The last knuckle of the middle finger is slightly bent, so that tips of the three longest fingers are even. Execute the jab with the same movements

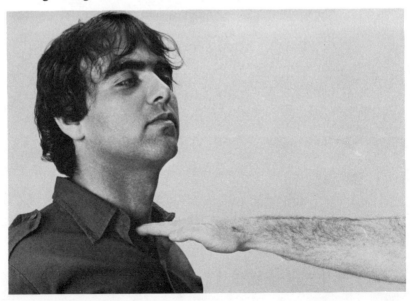

as the blow with a closed fist (see Exercise 8). This blow gains distance for the defender, and is a more accurate blow than a straight fist punch. Use it to attack vulnerable spots, such as the hollow of the throat, the eyes, or the groin.

3. *Heel of hand*—Fingers are slightly curled. The heel of the hand is the point of impact. This blow is especially effective to the base of the nose and to the chin. The heel of the hand is wider than the first two knuckles of a fist, and therefore it is easier to hit the target. This blow will stun the attacker. Execute it the same as Exercise 8.

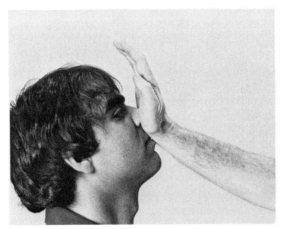

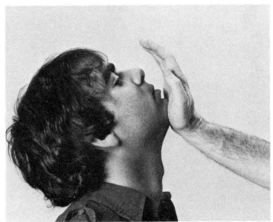

Exercise 12 Inward Horizontal Elbow Blow

1. Starting position.
2. Advance one step with left foot, fists at chest height. Push off with right foot, heel pointed outward. Turn to left and sweep elbow forward toward attacker's chin. Point of impact is the front bone of the elbow.

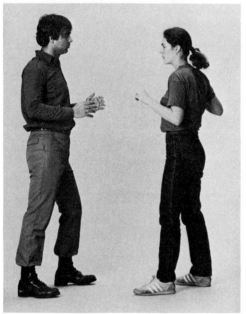

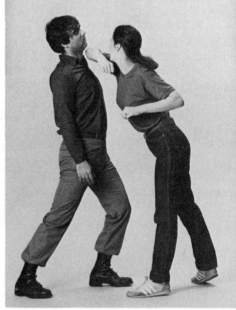

EXERCISE 13 UPWARD ELBOW BLOW

1. Starting position.
2. Advance one step with left foot; follow with right. Raise elbow to shoulder height, striking blow under attacker's chin in upward movement. Point of impact is front of elbow.

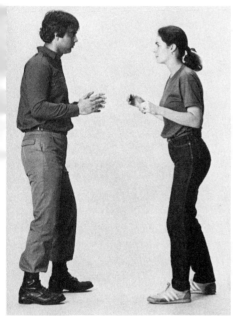

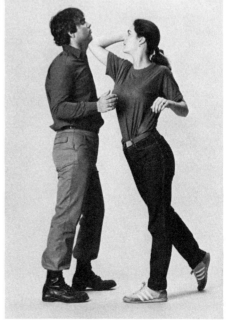

EXERCISE 14 VERTICAL DOWNWARD ELBOW BLOW

1. Starting position. Defender bends at trunk.
2. Advance with left foot, turn trunk in the direction of target. Raise right arm.
3. Bend knees as arm is brought down, striking attacker at the base of the skull or back. This blow can be used as a follow-up to Exercise 13.

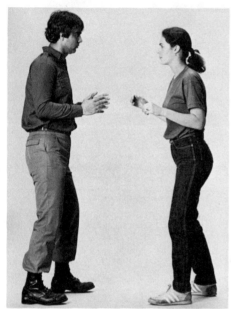

1

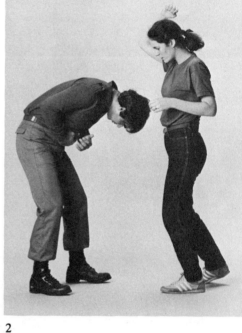

2

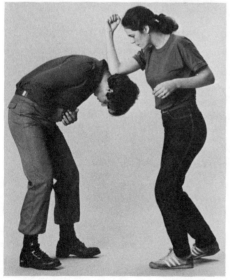

3

EXERCISE 15 BACKWARD ELBOW BLOW

1. Starting position.
2. Turn trunk to right, drawing elbow back to attacker's stomach.

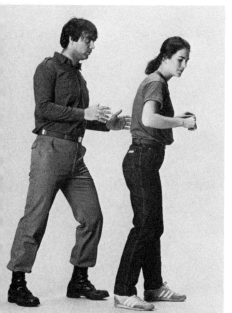

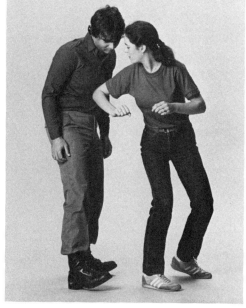

Exercise 16 Backward and Upward Elbow Blow

1. Starting position.
2. Bend trunk forward and draw right elbow vertically upward toward attacker's face, while turning to the right.

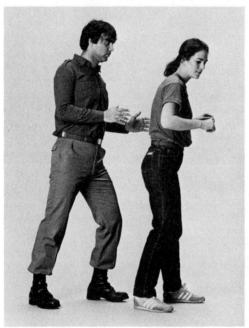
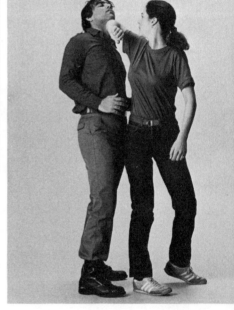

Kicks

IN KICKING, the leg is used as an effective tool for both offense and defense. The advantage of the kick over the blow is distance: To hit the opponent from as far away as possible to cause him severe injury.

An effective kick is a function of:

A. *Hardness*—Strong bones, army shoes, etc.

B. *Range*—The leg is longer than the arm.

C. *Strength*—Leg muscles are the largest and the strongest of the body.

D. *Accuracy from a distance*—The ability to hit vulnerable targets such as the ribs, kidneys, waist and hips, stomach, groin, thighs, shins, knees, ankles and spine.

Points to emphasize:

1. Practice the general movement first, then pick a spot on the wall, or a target, such as a corner of a table, and try to come as close as possible to striking it. Practice in front of a mirror to make sure you are performing the kick correctly. Once you can consistently strike your target, work on speed. Although the exercises are shown with a partner, practice them by yourself at first.

2. During the kick, the body weight shifts to the part of the foot that lands the kick.

3. Exercises show kicks with the right leg. For kicks with the left, follow the same movements, but use opposite arms and legs. Practice both right and left kicks.

EXERCISE 17 FOOT POSITIONS

The position of the foot during a kick depends on how far you are from your target.

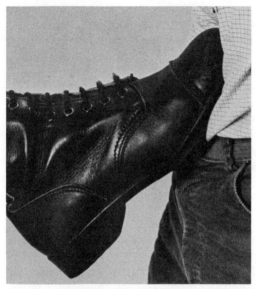

1. *Toe*—Used mainly in a front attack. Requires accuracy, momentum and distance. This is the least powerful kick, but can inflict injury.

2. *Sole of the foot*—The most powerful and most general. This position causes the least injury, and is used to push the attacker away.

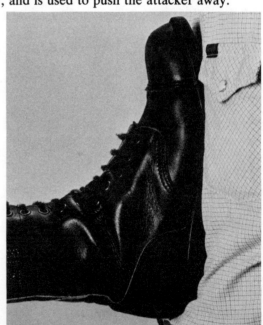

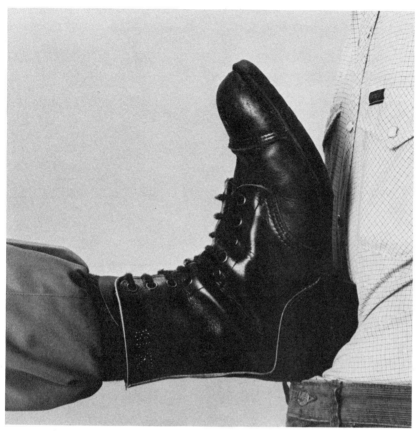

3. *Heel*—Requires the greatest accuracy and the least distance. It is stronger than a toe kick and will inflict injury, but is harder to deliver effectively.

Exercise 18 Defense Kick

1. Starting position.
2. Bend back, bend right leg, and kick left leg out, toe pointed.

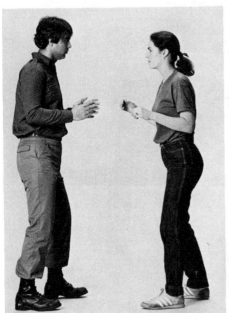

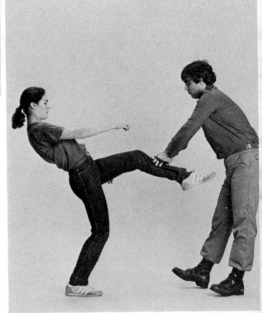

EXERCISE 19 OFFENSE KICK

1. Starting position.
2. Step slightly to the left with left foot.
3. Lean back, bend right leg, and raise left leg in kick to enemy's groin, toe pointed.

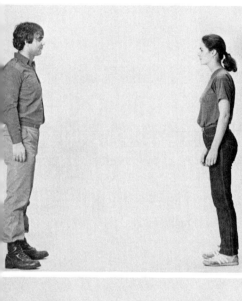

1

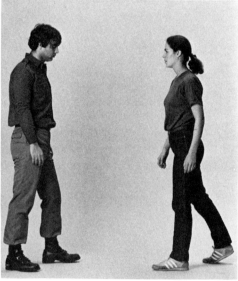

2

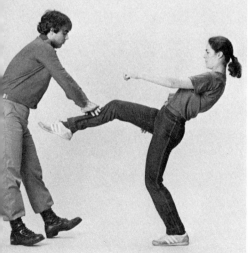

3

A PERSON UNDER ATTACK reacts by defending him or herself, whether the attack is sudden and isolated or part of a larger battle. Defense techniques include bodily evasion or deflecting or blocking the kick or blow.

Once you've become accurate and fast with the basic exercises in the preceding section, begin to work with a partner to improve your reaction and response.

Points to emphasize:

1. *Concentrate*—Be alert to the circumstances, to your surroundings, and to the manner of the attack. You will be better prepared to make an effective defense.
2. *Timing*—Execute the defense at the correct moment. Your reactions should surprise your opponent, so that he does not have time to prepare an effective defense.
3. *Defense and immediate attack*—will disable your attacker and prevent him or her from attacking again.
4. *Objective*—Avoid being struck.
5. *The more you practice, the better you'll become.*

EXERCISE 20 DEFENSE WITH RIGHT FOREARM AGAINST DIRECT BLOW

1. Starting position.
2. Turn trunk and forearm to the right and deflect blow with right forearm, palm toward body, hand clenched. Advance one step to the left.
3. Follow with upward left-fist blow.

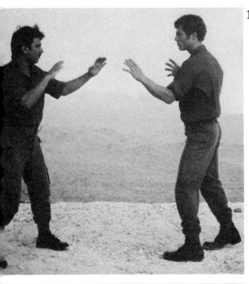

1

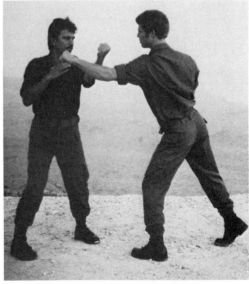

2

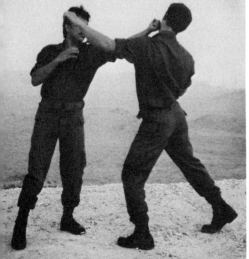

3

Exercise 21 Defense Against Direct Blow

1. Starting position.
2. Deflect attacker's right forearm near wrist with left hand. Advance with left foot, tilting head to the left.
3. Follow with right-fist blow to stomach.
4. Then with blow to groin.

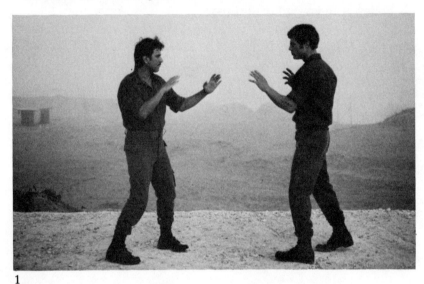

1

2

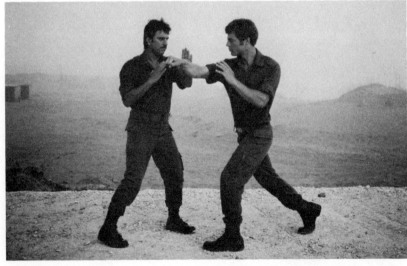

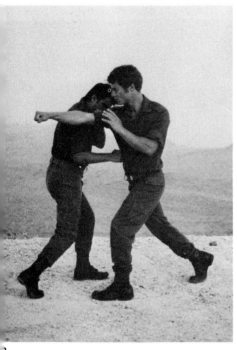

3

4

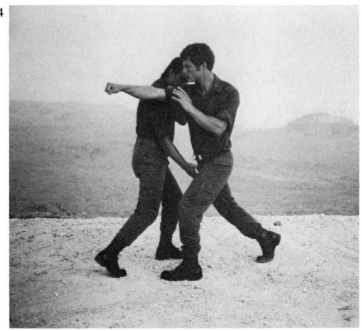

Exercise 22 Sideways Defense and Attack Against Direct Blow

1. Starting position.
2. Lean back, left hand above attacker's forearm.
3. As attacker strikes, bring left forearm over his right arm, pulling his arm down with wrist. Right hand strikes blow to attacker's chin.

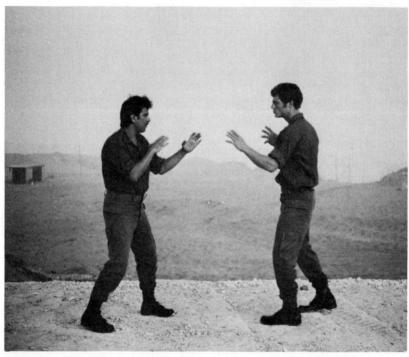

1

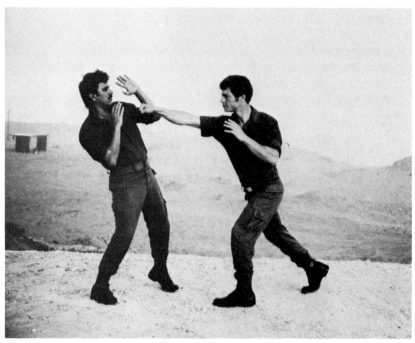

2

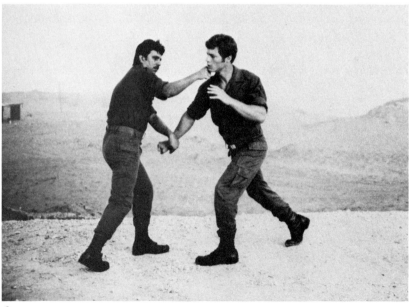

3

EXERCISE 23 DEFENSE AGAINST KICK AND BLOW

1. Starting position.
2. Step forward and slightly to the left with left foot. Turn body one quarter to the right as attacker kicks and prepares to throw a right punch to the face. Push attacker's leg to the right with left palm or

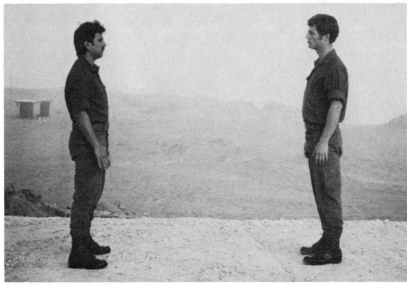

1

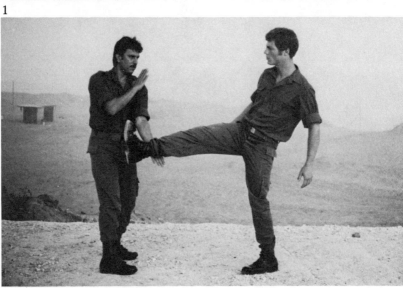

2

clenched fist. Move right hand toward left shoulder and deflect blow with forearm.

3. Pull attacker's right hand down; prepare to deliver blow to attacker's chin.
4. Grip attacker's right forearm with left hand; deliver blow with right fist to chin.

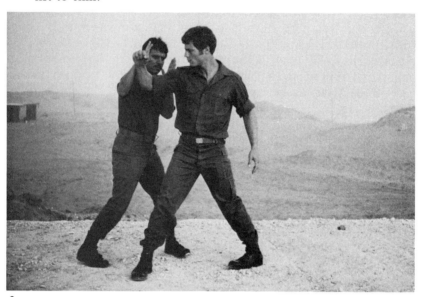

3

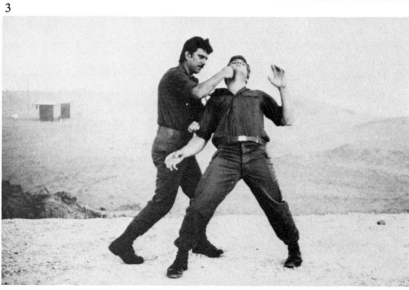

4

Grips and Releases

THIS SECTION COVERS the different exercises for grips and releases. Grips are used when blows or kicks are not possible or when a grip would be more efficient and effective, such as in close contact battles. These exercises also raise the fighter's self-confidence by enabling him or her to break the attacker's violent grip and to overcome him. Apart from an attacker's intention to cause injury, he might also be very strong. The release therefore must be resolute and quick to be effective.

A grip is an offense tactic, usually used when you don't want to injure the attacker, but you need to restrain him until help comes, or to lead him away. (See section on Policemen's Lead, page 174.) An effective grip depends on the strength in your hands and arms.

Points to emphasize:

1. Practice these exercises with a partner.
2. In order to release your hand or forearm, you must exploit the weakest part of the grip, usually the gap between the attacker's thumb and fingers, using your arm as a lever against the attacker's hand.
3. In open holds or holds in which your arms and hands are free, don't try to pull your attacker's hands apart. Try to pry just one finger out of the grip and bend it as far back as you can. This is usually enough to get him to release his grip.
4. If you are gripped or held, it is usually easier to get the attacker to release you himself by attacking a reachable part of his body, such as a stomp on the foot, a kick in the shin, a punch to the nose or the groin.

EXERCISE 24 OVERHAND GRIP AND RELEASE

1. Attacker's right hand grips defender's left arm.
2. Defender turns arm inward by pulling his hand toward the gap between the attacker's thumb and index finger, and at the same time,
3. pulls arm toward chest. Be sure to use the arm as a crowbar, twisting arm up while elbow points toward the attacker.

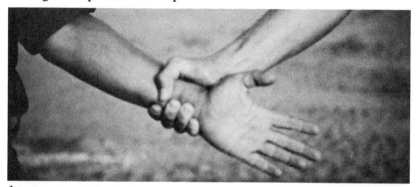

1

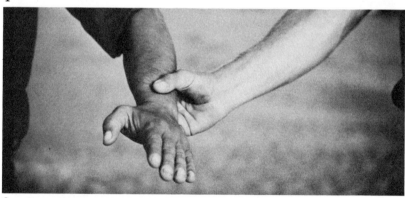

2

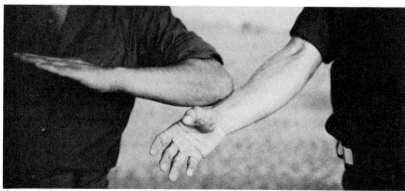

3

Exercise 25 Underhand Grip and Release

1. Starting position—Attacker's right hand grips defender's right hand.
2. Defender turns arm and hand out, directing hand toward the gap between the attacker's thumb and index finger, and
3. pulls arm toward his chest. The arm should be used as a lever against the top of the attacker's hand, elbow points toward attacker.

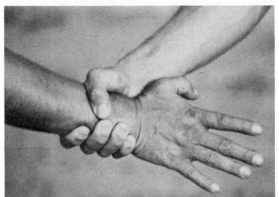

1

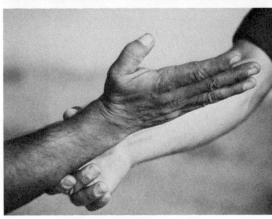

2

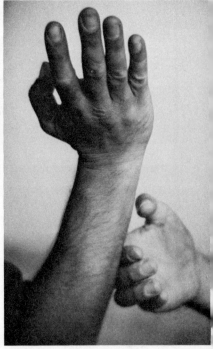

3

Exercise 26 Overhand Grip and Release

1. Starting position—Attacker's left hand grips defender's right hand.
2. Defender turns right hand and forearm inward, and using arm as a lever against the top of attacker's hand, pulls his forearm toward his own stomach. Defender releases hand through the gap between the attacker's thumb and index finger.

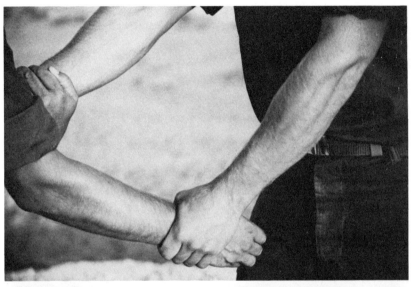

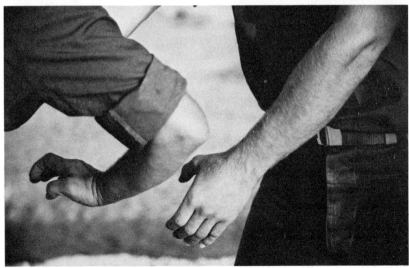

Exercise 27 Overhand Grip and Release of Two Hands

1. Starting position—Attacker grips defender's two arms at forearms and wrists.
2. Defender bends arms at elbows and draws forearms across chest.
3. Defender rotates arms outward, toward gaps between attacker's thumbs and index fingers, so that thumbs point out. Push elbows toward attacker while drawing forearms out to side (lever action against top of attacker's hands).

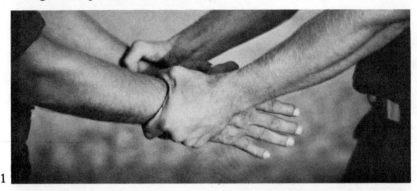

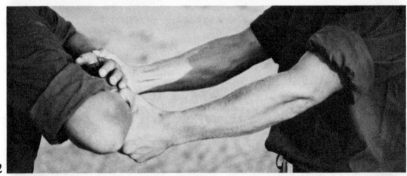

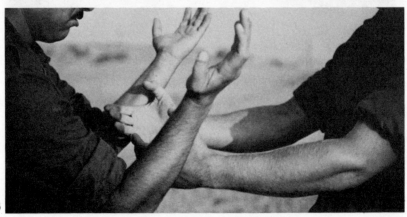

Exercise 28 Release from Underhand Grip on Two Hands While Prone

1. Starting position—Defender is pinned to the ground with knees bent. Attacker sits on his stomach, holding both hands down in underhand grip.
2. Defender pulls arms straight and up to slightly overhead position and lifts pelvis.
3. As attacker falls forward, defender punches him in the groin with a closed fist.

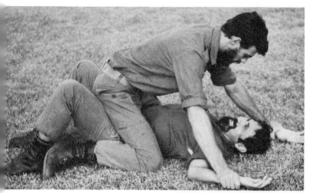

1

2

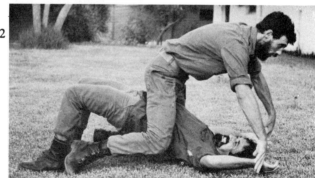

3

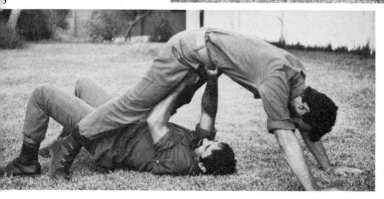

Exercise 29 Two-Handed Grip and Release

1. Starting position—Attacker grips defender's right arm in two-handed grip.

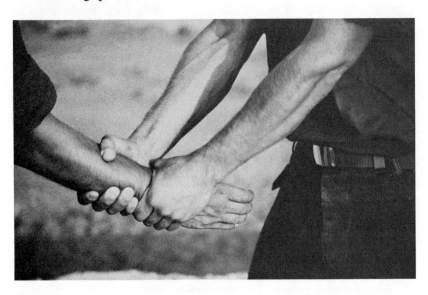

2. Defender inserts left hand between attacker's hands and grips his own right fist from below and in front.

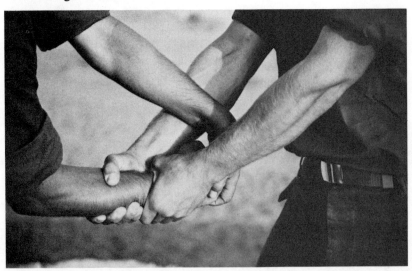

3. Defender pulls right fist up, toward attacker's elbow.

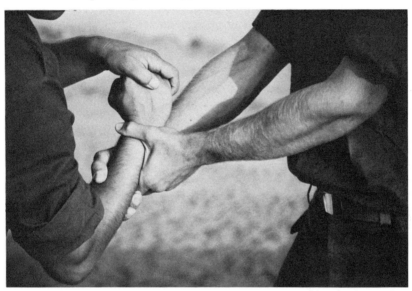

4. Defender pulls right fist abruptly to the left, forearm horizontal and elbow toward the attacker, and releases hand.

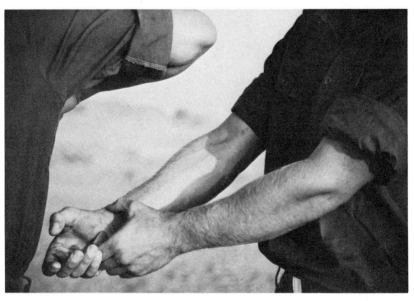

EXERCISE 30 ALTERNATIVE RELEASE FROM TWO-HANDED GRIP

1. Starting position—Attacker grips defender's right hand with two hands.
2. Defender closes fingers into tight fist and inserts left hand between attacker's forearms, gripping his own fist.
3. Defender pulls hands down and through attacker's grip, using an arm as lever against the tops of attacker's hands.

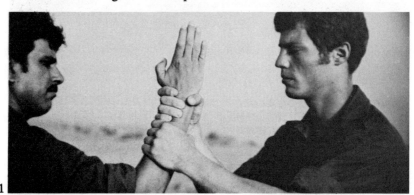

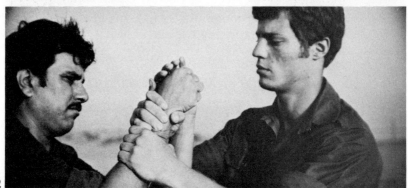

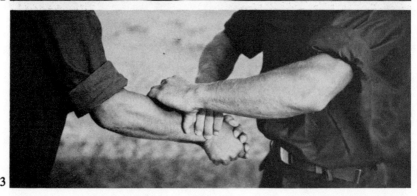

Exercise 31 Front Strangulation and Release

1. Starting position—Attacker stands in front of defender and grips defender's throat in two hands.
2. Defender pivots back on left foot and brings left arm up and over attacker's right arm, bending to right.
3. Defender lowers right arm, and with left arm, sweeps attacker's right arm down.
4. Defender turns to right and raises left elbow.
5. Defender follows up with upward elbow jab to attacker's chin.

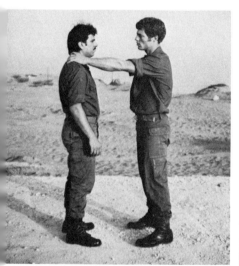

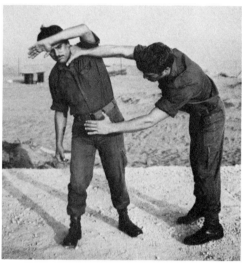

2

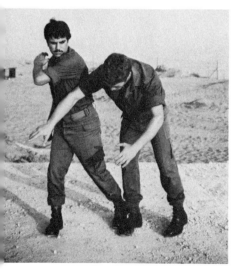

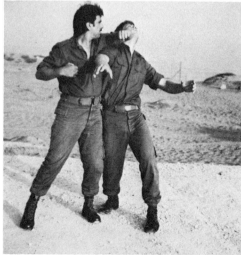

4

Exercise 32 Alternate Release from Front Strangulation

1. Starting position—Attacker faces defender and grips defender's throat in two hands.
2. Defender grips each of attacker's hands and pulls out to the side, while raising knee in kick to the groin.

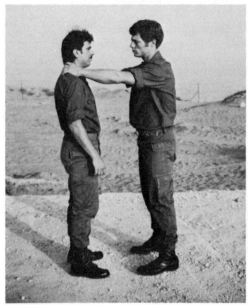

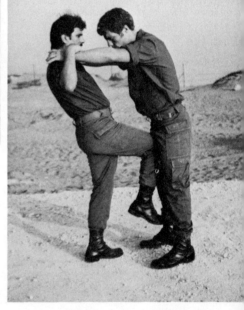

Exercise 33 Strangulation from Behind and Release

1. Starting position—Attacker stands behind defender and grips defender's neck with both hands.
2. Defender reaches back and grabs attacker's thumbs; fingers curl around attacker's thumbs.
   Pad of defender's thumb rests on knuckle of index finger.

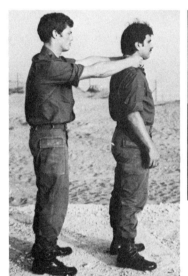
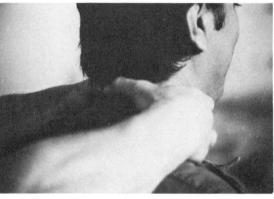

1

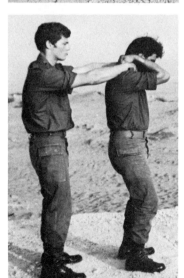
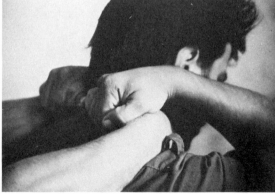

2

3. Defender pulls attacker's thumbs forward and out to the sides.
4. Then he releases attacker's right hand, takes one step back with left foot, and bends trunk forward.
5. Defender follows with the finger jab to groin or a backward elbow jab to the stomach.

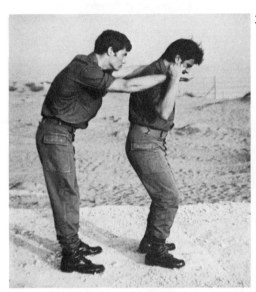

3

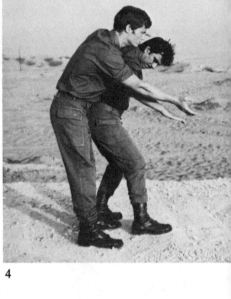

4

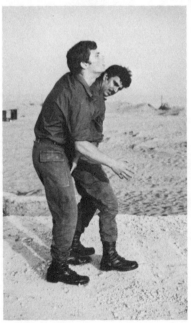

5

EXERCISE 34 STRANGULATION WHILE PRONE AND RELEASE

1. Starting position—Defender lies on back, knees bent, arms free. Attacker sits on defender's stomach and grips defender's throat with both hands.
2. Defender raises pelvis off ground while gripping attacker's hands and pulling them out to the side.
3. As attacker falls forward, defender punches him in the groin with a closed fist.

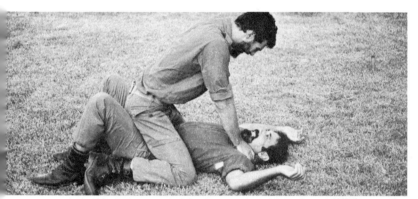

1

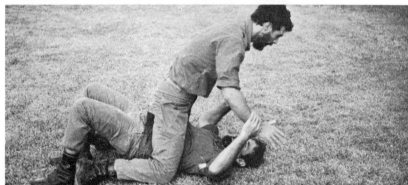

2

3

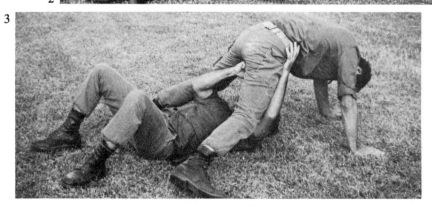

Exercise 35 Strangulation from the Side While Prone and Release

1. Starting position—Defender lies on back, knees bent, arms free. Attacker kneels to his right side, and grips defender's throat with both hands.
2. Defender jabs attacker's eyes with fingertips,
   or,
   defender punches attacker's chin with fist.

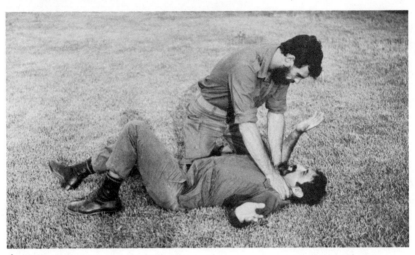

1

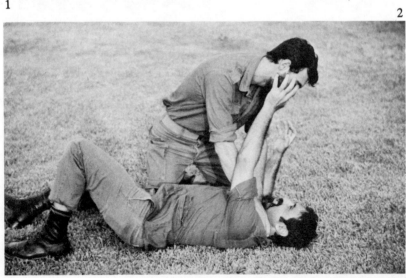

2

b

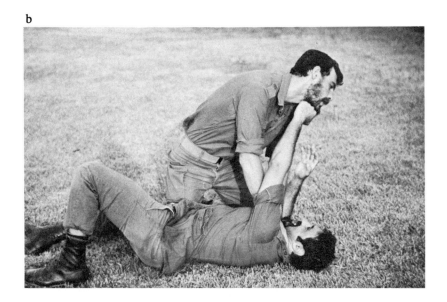

3. Defender grips attacker's hands and raises right knee against attacker's stomach.

3

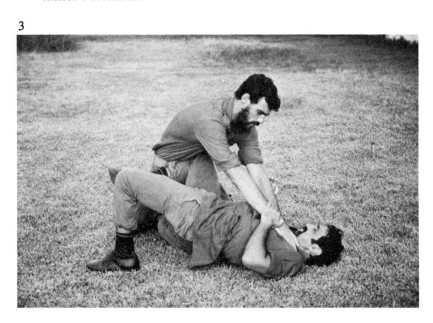

4. Defender lifts left leg and grips attacker's head between back of thigh and calf. Defender pulls attacker's left hand toward chin, in a two-handed grip.
5. Defender brings left leg, with attacker's head, down to the ground. Defender releases attacker's left hand, and grabs his right arm in a two-handed grip, then lifts pelvis and pulls attacker's arm down and to the right, breaking his elbow.

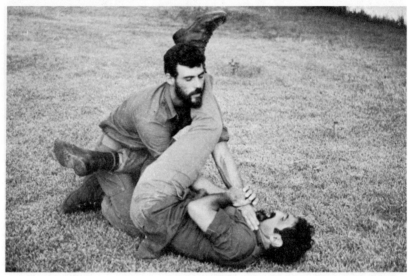

4

5

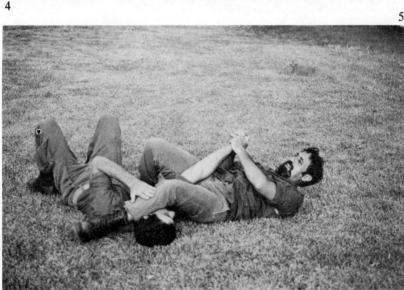

Exercise 36 Neck Grip from Behind and Release

1. Starting position—Attacker stands behind defender and grips defender's neck between right upper arm and forearm. Defender stands with arms slightly out from sides.
2. Defender grips attacker's right wrist in a two-handed grip.
3. Defender takes one step forward with right foot and pivots one-quarter back while bending forward and pulling attacker's right arm toward defender's diaphragm.

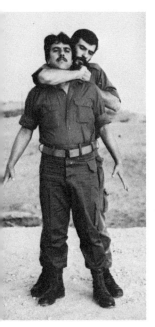

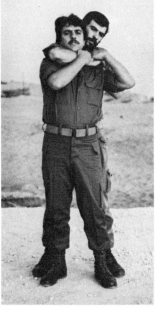

2

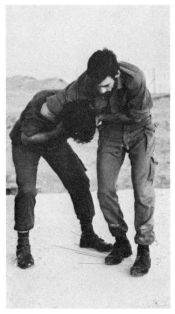

3

4. Defender continues to pivot back until release is completed. Defender grips attacker's right hand in defender's left hand. Defender's right hand grips attacker's right upper arm, and pulls attacker's arm behind his back.
5. Defender follows with toe kick or knee kick to attacker's face.

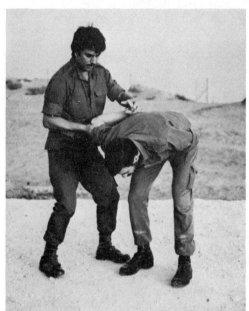

4

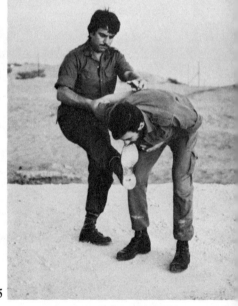

5

EXERCISE 37 FRONT NECK GRIP AND RELEASE

1. Starting position—Defender bends forward at the waist, knees slightly bent. Attacker grips defender's neck between arm and forearm.
2. Defender grips attacker's right wrist with his left hand, and with right hand, throws a fist punch to the attacker's groin.

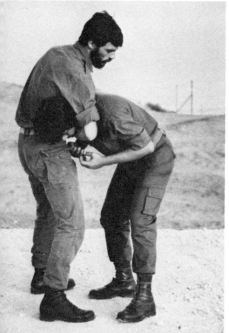

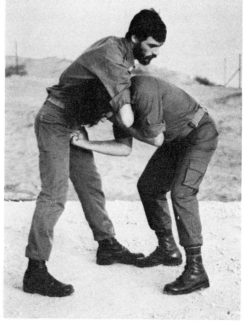

2

3. Defender steps forward with right foot and pivots back 180 degrees, pulling attacker's right arm out and back.
4. Defender pivots forward, facing the attacker, and delivers a knee kick to the groin.

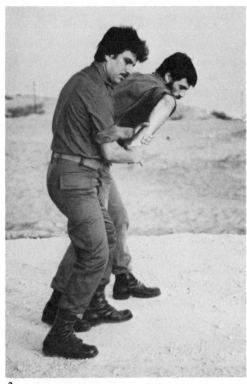

3

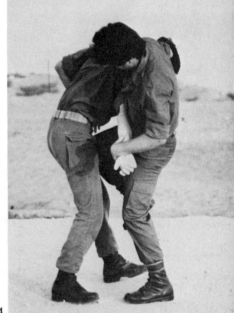

4

Exercise 38 Neck Grip from the Side and Release

1. Starting position—Defender stands with legs apart, bent forward from the waist and to the right. Attacker stands in front of defender and grips defender's neck between upper arm and forearm.
2. Defender bends forward and grabs attacker's groin with right hand. At the same time, the left hand reaches up and the middle finger pushes hard against the base of the attacker's nose, or

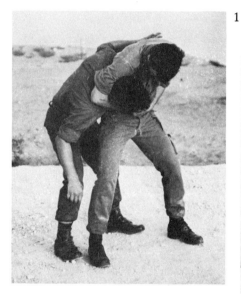

1

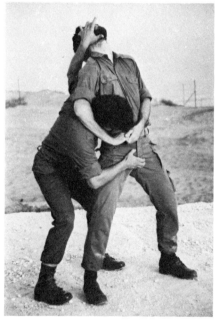

2

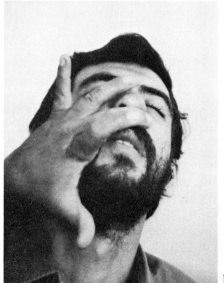

b

the middle finger jabs attacker's eye, or

three longest fingers push against attacker's jugular vein, or,

defender grabs attacker by the hair and pulls head back.

c

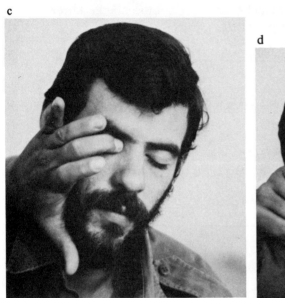

d

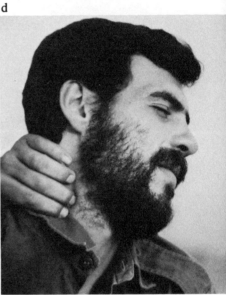

e

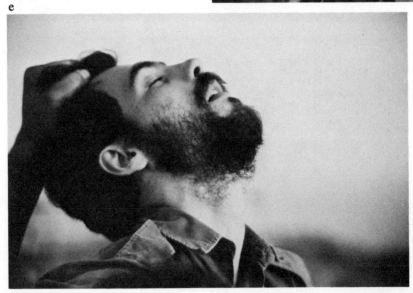

Exercise 39 Release from Head Grip While Prone

1. Starting position—Defender lies on back, knees bent, arms free. Attacker sits on ground, legs apart and bent at knees, right arm grips defender's neck between upper arm and forearm. Left hand holds defender's right upper arm.
2. Defender's hand pulls against the base of attacker's nose, pulling head back.
3. Right hand grabs attacker's groin.

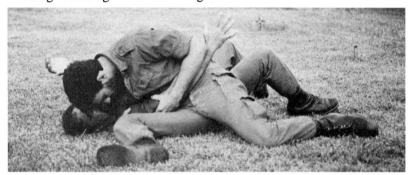

1

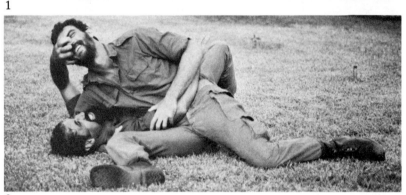

2

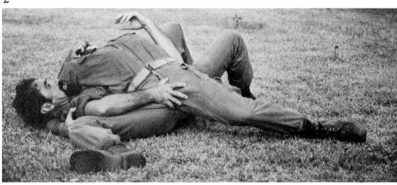

3

Exercise 40 Open Grip from Front and Release

1. Starting position—Defender stands with legs apart, arms out from sides. Attacker faces defender and grabs him around the waist.
2. Defender turns head and bites attacker's ear, or defender grabs attacker's hair with right hand and pulls down and to the right, while the left hand grabs attacker's chin and pulls it to the left, or defender jabs thumbs into attacker's eyes, or
defender pushes thumbs into the base of attacker's nose, pushing his head back.

1

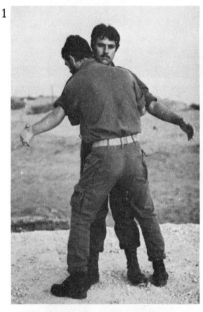

2

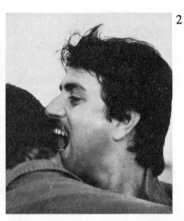

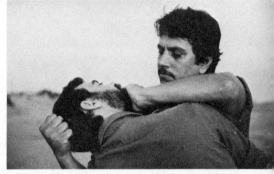

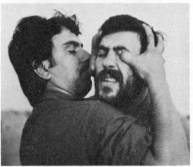

c

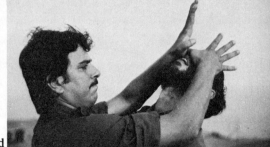

d

Exercise 41 Alternate Release from Open Front Grip

1. Starting position—Defender stands with legs apart, arms free. Attacker, bent at the waist, grips defender around the waist.
2. Defender raises knee and delivers a kick to the groin and immediately
3. follows with a toe kick to attacker's shin.
4. As attacker falls forward, defender delivers a downward elbow blow to the back of his neck.

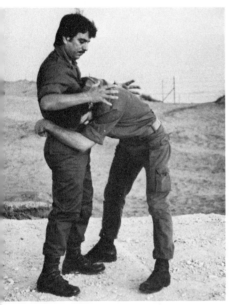

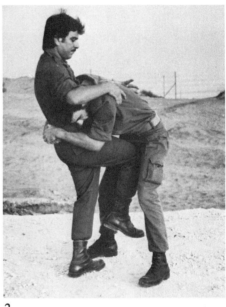

2

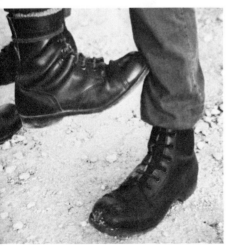

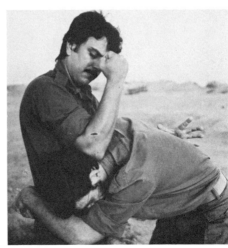

3

4

EXERCISE 42 OPEN GRIP FROM BEHIND AND RELEASE

1. Starting position—Defender stands with legs apart and arms free and slightly out from the sides.
2. Defender bends trunk forward and grips attacker's hands. Body weight shifts to the left foot as defender looks toward attacker's feet and kicks attacker's shin with right heel.
3. Defender pries one finger from attacker's grip and bends finger back.

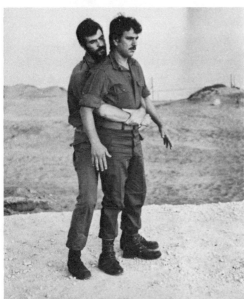

1

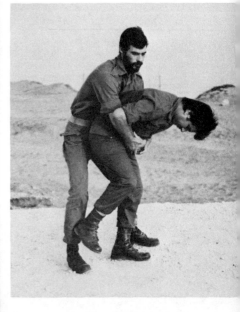

2

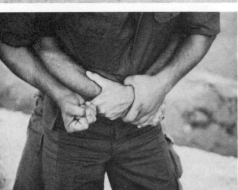

3

4. Defender continues to bend finger back until attacker turns. Defender turns toward attacker and
5. follows with toe kick to groin.

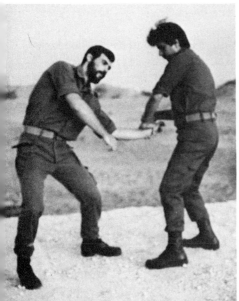
4

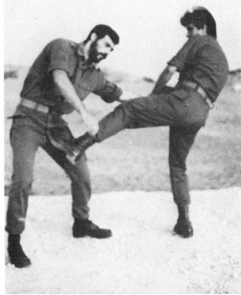
5

EXERCISE 43 CLOSED FRONT GRIP AND RELEASE

1. Starting position—Defender stands straight, legs slightly apart, arms pinned to sides. Attacker grabs defender around arms and waist.
2. Defender moves pelvis back and delivers finger jab to attacker's groin.
3. As attacker pulls back, defender raises knee and delivers knee kick to groin, or defender kicks attacker's shin with inside of heel.

1

2

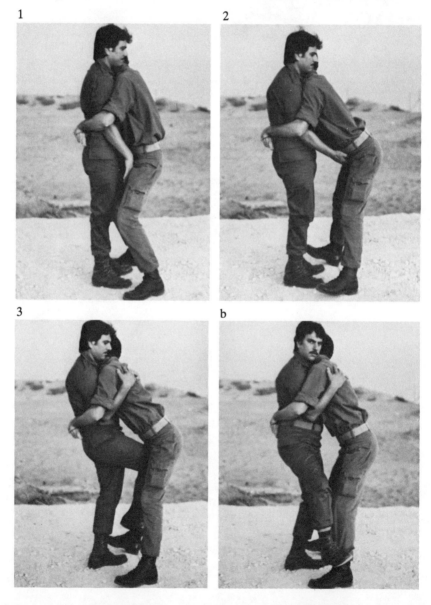

3

b

EXERCISE 44 CLOSED GRIP FROM BEHIND AND RELEASE

1. Starting position—Defender stands with arms pinned to sides and legs slightly apart. Attacker grips defender around arms and waist from behind.
2. Defender pushes head back, hitting attacker in the face.
3. Defender bends forward and delivers finger jab to attacker's groin. Attacker will draw pelvis back.
4. Defender delivers a heel kick to attacker's shin.

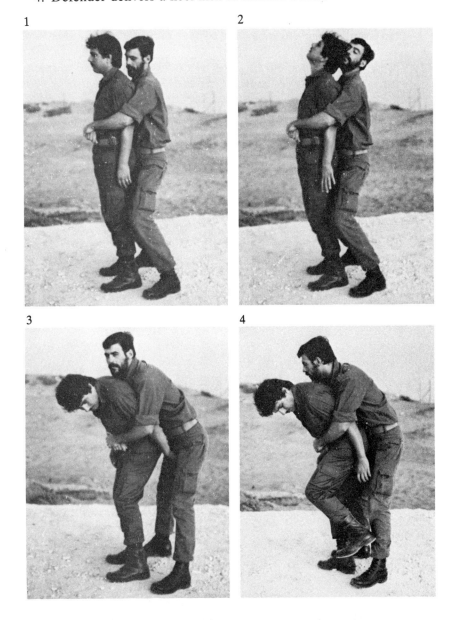

Throws

THROWS ARE OFFENSIVE MOVES, executed to gain advantage over one's opponent. They are essential in face-to-face combat.

Points to emphasize:

1. Practice these with a partner. Try to take him by surprise.
2. Concentrate on performing the correct movement first, then on speed and accuracy.
3. Throws *must* be done quickly, very accurately, and without warning your opponent in order to be effective.

EXERCISE 45 MOWING

1. Starting position—Opponents stand face to face.

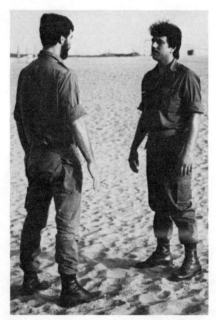

1

2. Attacker steps forward and slightly to the left, with left foot 8 inches beyond defender's right foot. Attacker shifts defender's weight to his right foot by gripping defender's right arm and pulling down and back in the direction of the fall.
3. Attacker simultaneously strikes blow to defender's chin with the heel of his right hand.

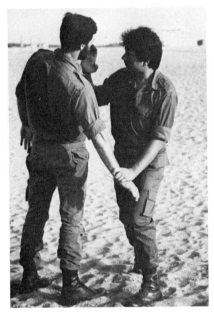

2

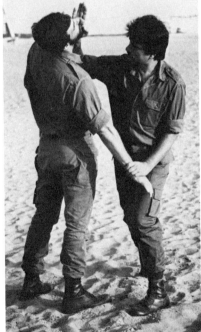

3

4. Attacker brings right leg behind defender's right leg, and turns foot inward.
5. Attacker draws right leg straight back and up, sweeping (mowing) defender's right leg with it, causing him to fall backward.
6. Attacker grips defender's right wrist with two hands, and delivers a kick with the right heel at defender's ribs or temple.

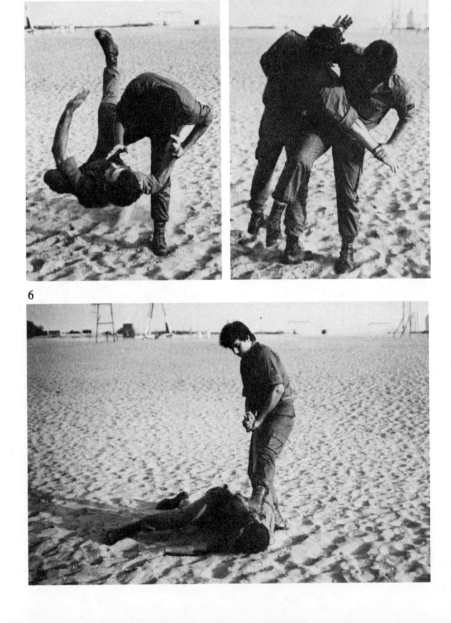

EXERCISE 46 SHIRT THROW

1. Starting position—Opponents face each other, arms at sides, legs slightly apart.
2. Attacker steps forward and slightly to the left, so that his foot is between attacker's feet, and grips defender's shirt collar with both hands, right hand slightly lower than the left.
3. Attacker quickly leaps and turns about face to the left. Attacker pushes rear toward defender's pelvis until knees are bent slightly. Attacker bends trunk forward slightly, then leans forward and spreads knees, pulling shirt and swinging defender overhead.

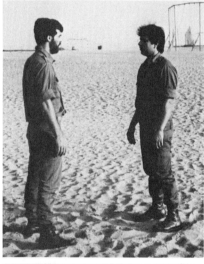

1

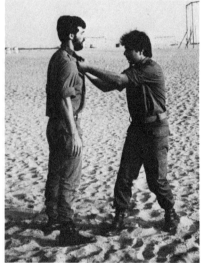

2

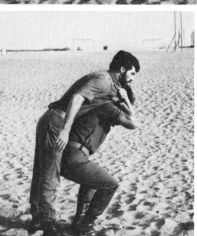

3

4. Attacker pushes his rear toward defender's stomach and raises defender on back, flipping him over.
5. Attacker follows with a kick to defender's face.

4

b

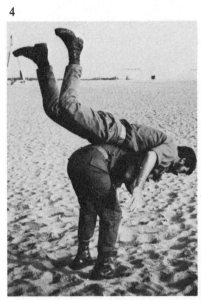
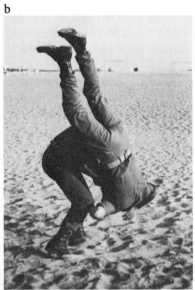

5

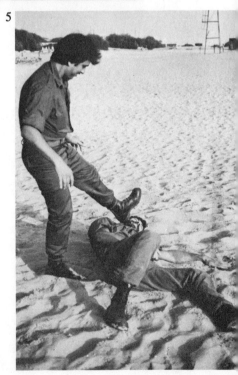

Exercise 47 "Self-Sacrifice"

1. Starting position—Opponents stand face to face, legs slightly apart.
2. Attacker steps toward defender with left foot, and grabs defender's shirt collar with both hands. If defender pushes, attacker grips defender's sleeves above the elbow.
3. Attacker drops to sitting position and plants right foot in defender's stomach above the groin.
4. Attacker rolls to back position, thrusting defender upward and backward with right leg. Simultaneously, attacker pulls defender's arms backward toward attacker's head.

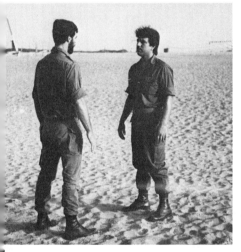

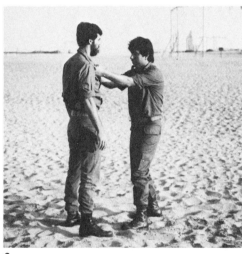

2

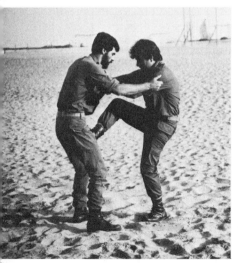

3

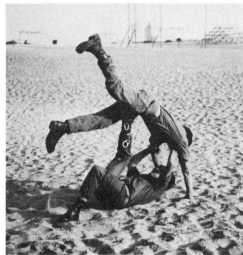

4

5. Attacker rises and turns toward defender.
6. Attacker runs to defender.
7. Attacker kicks defender in ribs.

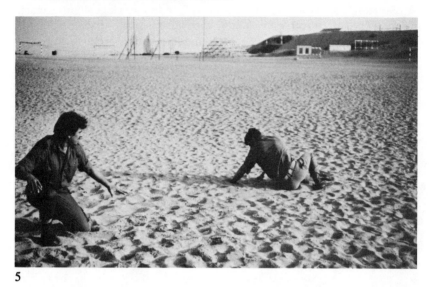

5

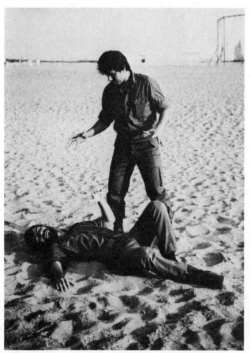

6

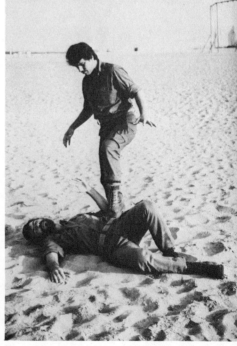

7

Defense from Attack with a Weapon

A WEAPON GIVES the attacker an advantage. The defender must first be thoroughly familiar with all the possible uses of a weapon in order to anticipate the attacker's moves and to respond with an adequate defense.

Points to emphasize:

In defending yourself against a weapon, remember to:
1. Notice the type of weapon and the way it is held by the attacker.
2. Concentrate on the attacker's movements—the directions he moves in and the way he handles the weapon.
3. Notice how quick your attacker is.
4. Time the defense precisely. Execute your defense as quickly as possible. You must be able to surprise the attacker; it will give you an advantage.
5. Any defense requires practice. Try these exercises with a partner, using sticks for the knives and toy guns for the pistols, while you gain proficiency.

Knives

EXERCISE 48 TYPICAL KNIFE GRIPS

1. *Regular grip*—The knife is held tight in an overhand grip, thumb overlaps index finger, with blade perpendicular to ground and the cutting edge up.

    This grip is used at a close distance and is the strongest grip, but the range of movement is narrow.

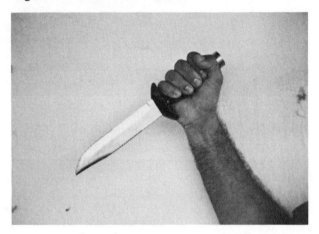

2. *Oriental grip*—The knife is held with fingers close on handle with thumb gripping the last joint of the index finger. The blade is perpendicular to the ground, the cutting edge down.

    This grip is used at a moderate distance. The Oriental grip is also a strong grip, but not as strong as the regular grip. It, too, gives the attacker a narrow range of movement.

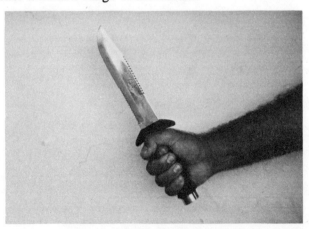

3. *Straight grip*—The butt of the knife handle rests in the heel of the hand in a modified overhand grip: The thumb is extended on the side of the handle; the index finger is directly below the thumb; other fingers curl around the handle. The blade is horizontal and parallel to the ground.

   The attacker gains greater distance with this grip. The straight grip is the weakest knife grip, but it gives the attacker the greatest flexibility and the widest range.

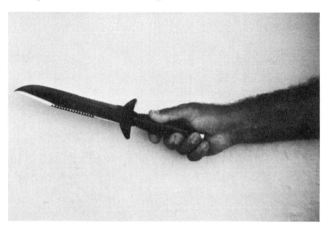

4. *Tearing grip or modified overhand grip*—The thumb is extended on the handle just behind the blade; index finger directly under thumb; remaining fingers curl around handle. Blade is vertical.

   This grip is used at medium range, but affords more distance than the Oriental grip. The tearing grip is weaker than the regular or Oriental grips, but is stronger than the straight grip while giving the attacker the same flexibility and wide range.

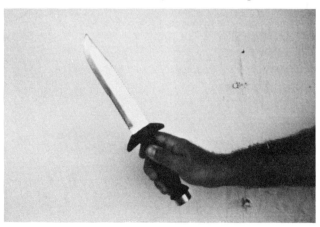

EXERCISE 49 DEFENSE AGAINST KNIFE IN REGULAR GRIP

1. Starting position—Defender stands with arms down and slightly out from the sides, feet slightly apart. Attacker stands in front of defender, legs slightly apart, holding knife in regular grip, elbow of other hand close to waist, forearm and hand in front. Attacker advances from a distance of about 8 feet.
2. Defender steps forward and slightly to the left with the left foot.
3. Defender delivers an attack kick to attacker's groin.
4. Defender follows with a hammer blow to the base of attacker's skull.

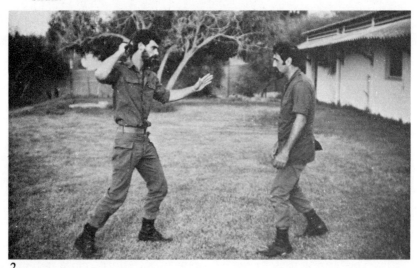

2

3

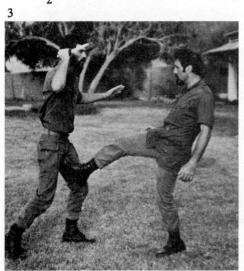

4

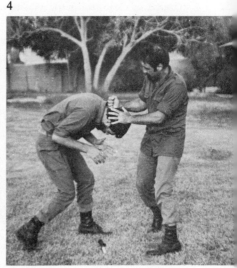

EXERCISE 50 DEFENSE AGAINST KNIFE HELD IN ORIENTAL GRIP

1. Starting position—Defender stands with legs slightly apart, arms at sides. Attacker faces the defender, knife held in Oriental grip, legs slightly apart, free arm at waist height and in front.
2. Defender steps forward and slightly to the left with the left foot. As attacker stabs, defender turns body one-quarter to the right, so that knife is in front. Defender pulls attacker's arm down with the outside of left forearm, and strikes a blow to the attacker's chin with right fist.

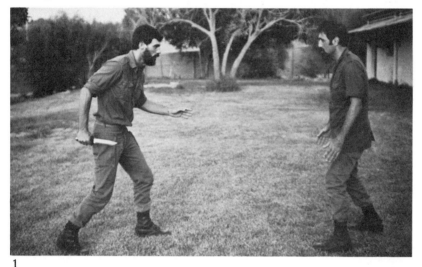

1

2

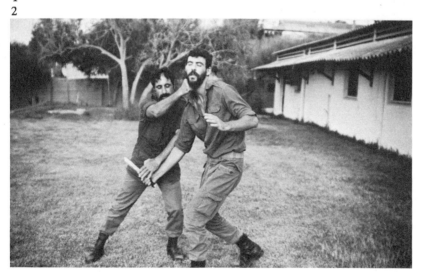

3. Defender grips attacker's right hand and turns it down and to the outside.
4. Defender maintains grip on attacker's right hand and delivers a kick to the groin.

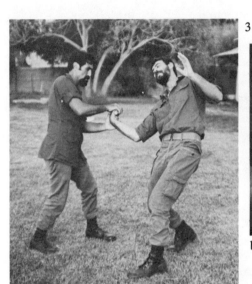

3

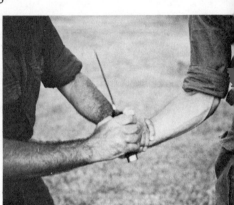

b

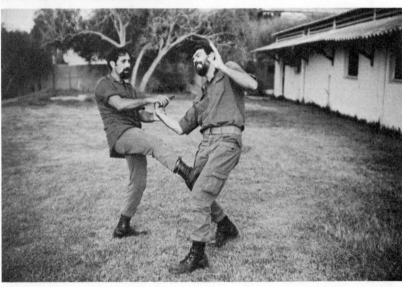

4

5. Defender keeps turning attacker's hand down and to the outside, forcing him to the ground. Defender follows with a stomp on the diaphragm.
6. Defender follows with a stomp to the temple or face, or a kick to the ribs with the left foot, while removing knife from the attacker's hand.

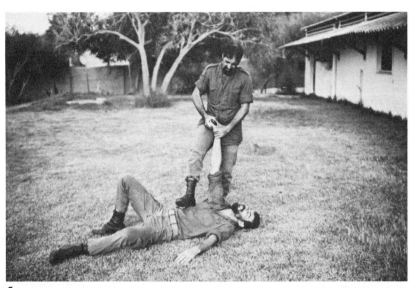

5

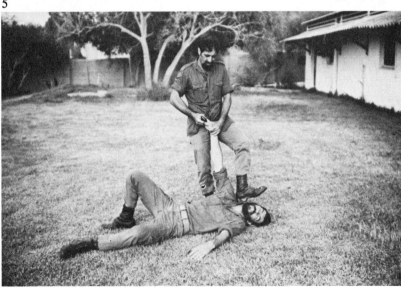

6

EXERCISE 51 DEFLECTION DEFENSE AGAINST DIRECT STAB WITH STRAIGHT GRIP OR TEARING GRIP

1. Starting position—Defender is in regular starting position (see Exercise 1). Attacker holds knife in straight grip or tearing grip, legs apart, other hand out in front at chest height.
2. As attacker advances and stabs, defender steps forward and to the left with the left foot, then pivots back one-quarter so that knife is in front. Defender pushes attacker's right arm (arm with knife) down with left forearm.
3. Defender grips attacker's sleeve with left arm and punches attacker's chin with a right fist.

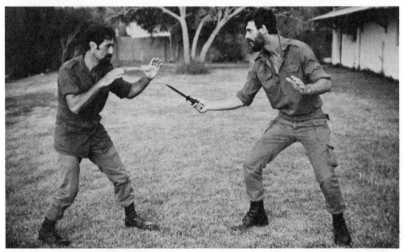

1

2

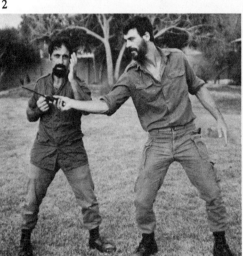

3

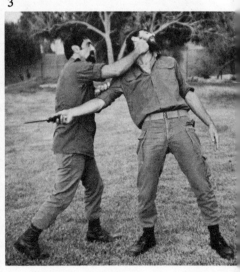

Exercise 52 Defense with Knife Against Knifing with Regular and Oriental Grips

1. Starting position—Defender stands with legs slightly apart, knife held in straight grip in right hand beside or slightly behind right leg. Attacker stands with legs apart, left leg slightly in front; knife held in regular (or Oriental) grip in right hand, left hand extended in front at chest height.
2. As attacker advances, the defender pivots one-quarter on right foot, right heel pointed out, and shifts body weight to right foot. Defender simultaneously raises right arm, with knife held in straight grip, and delivers a straight jab at attacker's throat.

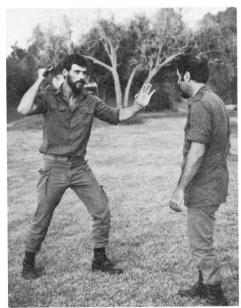

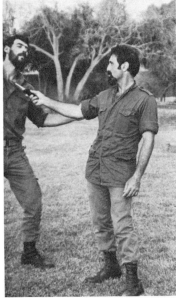

Clubs or Sticks

EXERCISE 53 DEFENSE WITH HAND ON THE OUTSIDE AGAINST CLUB

1. Starting position—Defender stands straight, legs slightly apart, arms at sides. Attacker stands to left of defender, legs apart, left foot forward, club in right hand, ready to strike.
2. As attacker advances and strikes, defender advances with left foot and deflects attacker's blow with back of left forearm against back of attacker's forearm.

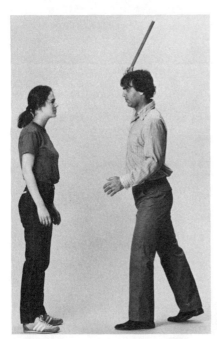

1

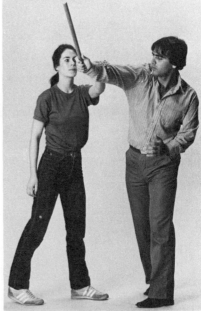

2

3. Defender simultaneously turns one-quarter to the right, forcing attacker's forearm down with the right hand and gripping attacker's sleeve with the left.
4. Defender follows with a right punch to the chin.

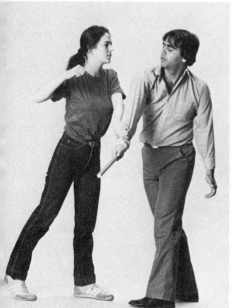

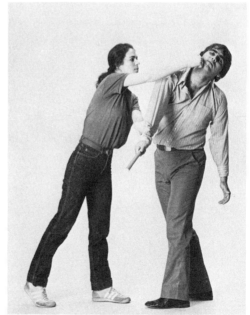

4

EXERCISE 54 DEFENSE WITH HAND ON THE INSIDE AGAINST CLUB

1. Starting position—Defender stands with legs slightly apart, facing attacker, arms down at sides. Attacker stands with legs apart, left foot forward, right arm raised with club.
2. As attacker advances toward defender and is about to strike, defender steps forward with left foot, raising left hand to the left. Defender must get as close as possible to attacker. Defender slides

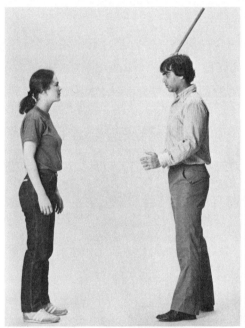

1

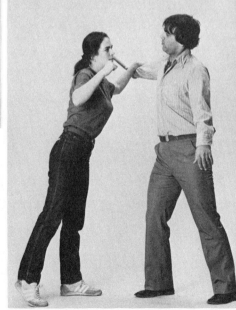

2

the back of his/her left forearm against the attacker's right forearm and punches attacker's chin with right fist.
3. Defender then delivers a knee kick to the groin.

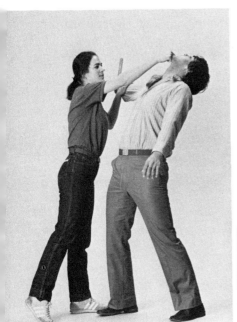

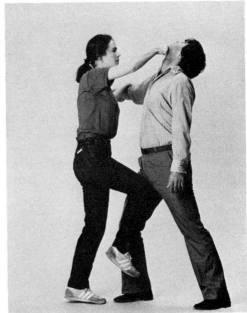

4

Guns

EXERCISE 55 DEFENSE AGAINST PISTOL THREAT FROM THE FRONT

1. Starting position—Defender stands with legs slightly apart, hands at sides. Attacker stands with legs slightly apart, right foot forward, pistol aimed at defender's chest.
2. Defender grabs barrel and butt of pistol in overhand grip, forcing the barrel down. Turn trunk about 45 degrees to the right. Defender leans forward, body weight on pistol, right hand in a fist, ready to punch.

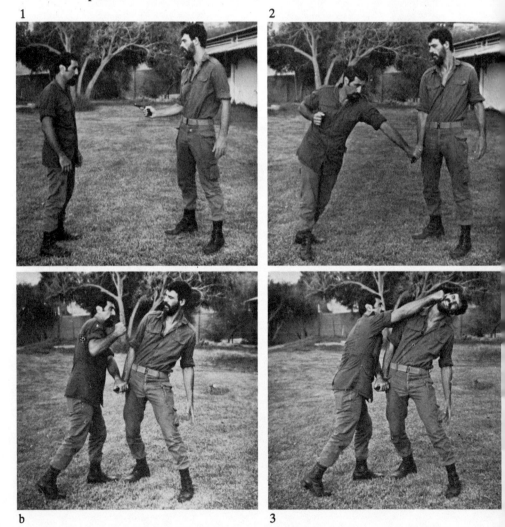

1

2

b

3

As the defender grabs the pistol, he presses on the attacker's trigger finger. The weapon will discharge, causing a finger burn. Regardless, the defender MUST NOT let go of the pistol.

3. Right hand delivers punch to the attacker's chin.
4. Defender's free hand grips the gun from below, fingers closed on the pistol hammer.
5. Defender turns pistol with both hands; barrel now points to the left.
6. Defender removes pistol from attacker's hand and draws a safe distance (about 6 feet) away.

4

5

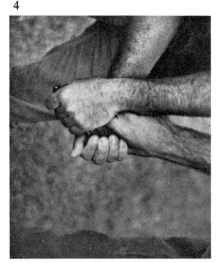
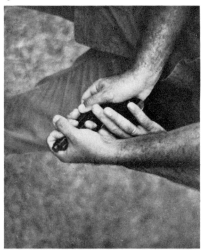

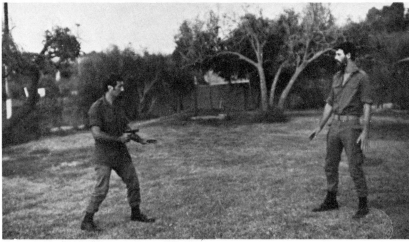

6

EXERCISE 56 DEFENSE AGAINST PISTOL THREAT FROM BEHIND

Note: Concentration is very important in this exercise; you must deduce which hand is holding the gun. If your attacker is standing more to the left, chances are he's holding the gun in his right hand. If he's standing more to the right, the gun is probably in his left. Use your peripheral vision to notice which hand is free. The other hand will have the gun.

1. Starting position—Defender stands straight, legs slightly apart, arms at sides. Attacker stands behind defender, legs slightly apart, pistol pointed at defender's back.
2. Defender pivots back on right foot, left arm raised to the side, pushing threatening hand out.

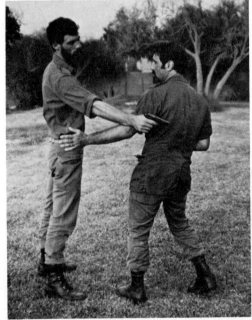

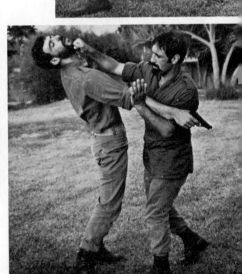

1

2

3

3. Defender grips attacker's arm between upper arm and forearm, and punches attacker in the chin with right fist.
4. Defender turns to the left, takes pistol in right hand with overhand grip and pulls it out of attacker's hand.
5. Defender delivers a blow to the attacker's temple with the butt of the pistol, or,

   after fist punch, defender delivers an inward horizontal elbow blow to the attacker's chin.
6. Defender follows with a knee kick to the groin and then removes pistol from attacker's hand.

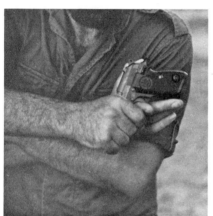

4

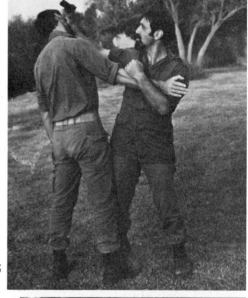

5

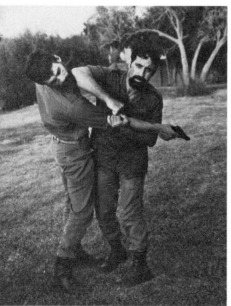

6

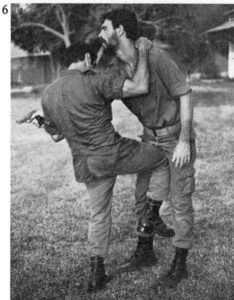

EXERCISE 57 DEFENSE AGAINST PISTOL THREAT FROM THE SIDE

1. Starting position—Defender stands with legs slightly apart, arms at sides. Attacker stands with legs slightly apart, and to the side of the defender, pistol aimed at defender's ribs, in front of defender's left arm.
2. Defender steps toward attacker with left foot and turns to the left so that pistol is in front. Defender's right hand grabs pistol barrel in underhand grip; defender's left grabs attacker's right arm at the wrist in an underhand grip.

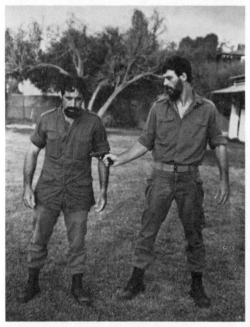

1

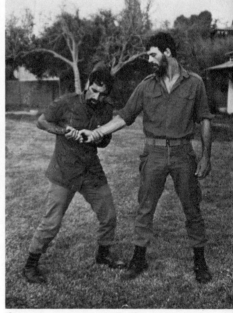

2

3. Defender pushes barrel toward opponent with the help of his right shoulder, until attacker releases gun,
4. and simultaneously delivers knee kick to the groin.
5. Defender then delivers blow to the attacker's temple with the butt of the gun.

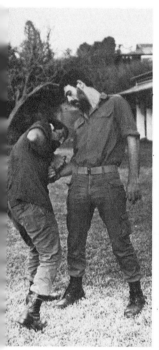

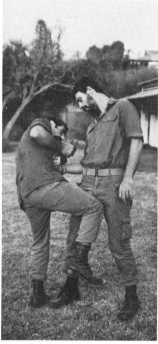

4

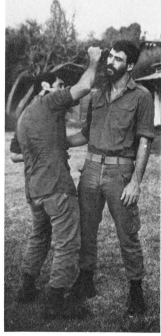

5

Policemen's Lead and Release

POLICEMEN'S LEAD EXERCISES enable a fighter to overcome his opponent and walk him away without causing severe injury. These exercises are especially useful for policemen, hence their name.

The principles involved in the policemen's lead are leverage against the elbow and a firm grip. The grip lead must be firm, quick, strong and accurate to prevent any escape or attack by the captive.

Points to emphasize:

1. The policemen's lead is used to capture someone without injuring them.
2. Use the crowbar principle—leverage against a joint—to discourage movement by the captive. If he moves, he'll create pain or self-injury.
3. The principle for the release is to sacrifice yourself momentarily, to put yourself at a disadvantage, in order to gain the advantage later.
4. During the release, your movements must be very fast. Surprise is the key element, it forces the captor to make a mistake and release his grip. Without surprise, you probably won't gain release, and will probably injure yourself.
5. Concentrate on perfecting the movement first, then on speed and accuracy.
6. Practice with a partner. Try to overcome him before he can overcome you.
7. During practice, be careful not to break your opponent's arm.
8. Be aware of the surprise element for the release and don't let go of your captive—no matter what.
9. The policemen's lead can be used to end a fight.

EXERCISE 58 POLICEMEN'S LEAD WITH LEVER

1. Starting position—Opponents are face to face, legs slightly apart, arms at sides.
2. Captor steps forward with left foot, about 6 inches away from prisoner's right foot, toes aligned with prisoner's toes. Captor's right hand grabs prisoner's right arm in underhand grip, and captor's left hand is ready to strike.
3. Captor pivots backward on left foot until he is standing side by side with prisoner. Captor strikes blow to right side of prisoner's chin. Captor raises prisoner's right arm up until it is straight out from the shoulder.

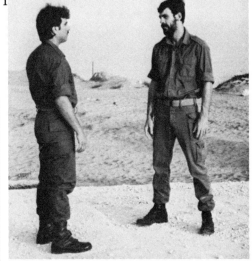

1

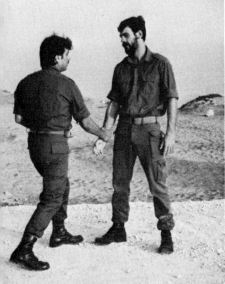

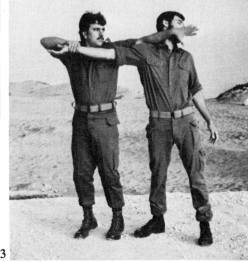

3

4. Captor grips prisoner's raised arm between his left upper arm and forearm. Captor grips the front of his shirt with the left hand.
5. Captor turns prisoner's hand farther to the right and pushes down on wrist to create lever against prisoner's elbow.

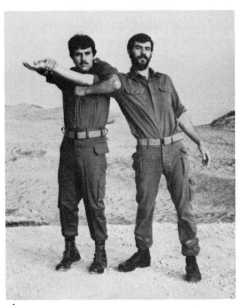

4

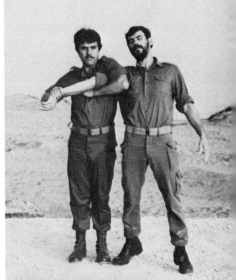

5

b

EXERCISE 59 RELEASE FROM POLICEMEN'S LEAD WITH LEVER

1. Starting position—Policemen's lead with lever (see Exercise 58).
2. Prisoner eases pressure on gripped arm by rising onto the balls of his feet. Prisoner coordinates his steps with those of his captor.
3. Prisoner shifts right foot before captor's left foot and leans against captor with his shoulder. Prisoner bends right arm at elbow and draws his arm to the left, his thumb points toward his right foot; prisoner's forearm presses against captor's forearm and prisoner's upper arm presses against captor's upper arm. Prisoner shifts body weight onto captor's arm, causing him to fall.

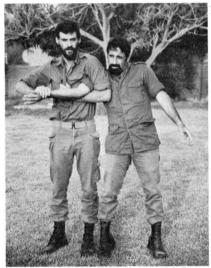

1

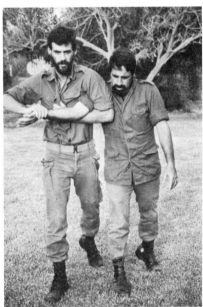

2

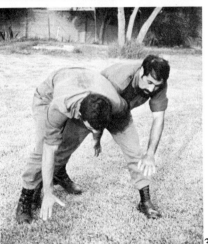

3

4. Prisoner falls with captor, extending legs back, and resting on toes.
5. Prisoner grips captor's left sleeve above elbow, pinning his arm to the ground. Prisoner rises to kneeling position, weight on right knee, adjacent to captor's arm. Prisoner bends captor's forearm and hand toward back.
6. Prisoner brings left foot against captor's arm above the elbow, releases grip on sleeve; pulls head back by the hair.

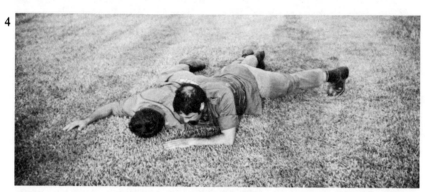

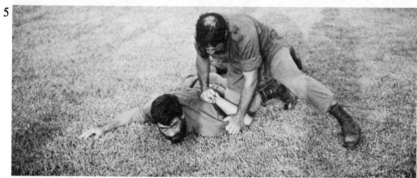

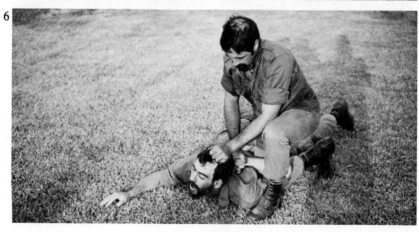

EXERCISE 60 POLICEMEN'S LEAD WITH FOREARM DRAWN BACK

1. Starting position—Captor and prisoner stand facing each other, arms at sides, legs slightly apart.
2. Captor steps forward and out with left foot, 4 inches away from prisoner's right foot. Captor grips prisoner's shirt above right elbow with right hand. Captor grips prisoner's knuckles and back of hand with left hand, fingers pointed down.

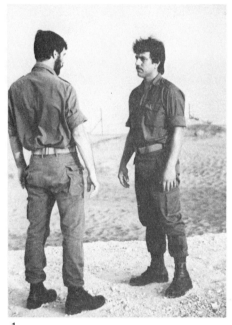

1

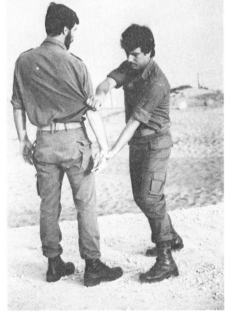

2

3. Captor pulls prisoner's shirt and raises prisoner's right arm behind back, bending hand toward elbow. Keep prisoner's elbow close to his body.
4. Captor releases prisoner's sleeve and grips his hair, pulling prisoner's head toward his elbow.

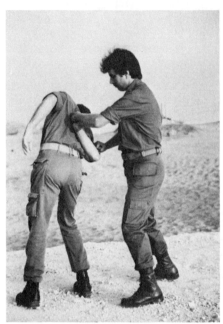

3

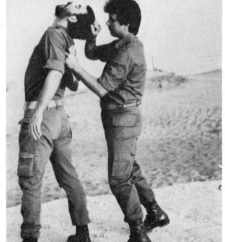

4

Exercise 61 Release from Policemen's Lead with Forearm Drawn Back

1. Starting position—Prisoner stands in front of captor. Captor grips prisoner's hair in right hand. Captor's left hand grips prisoner's right hand behind prisoner's back, and pulls up (see Exercise 60).
2. Prisoner bends forward and forcefully straightens arm. Captor steps back with left foot.

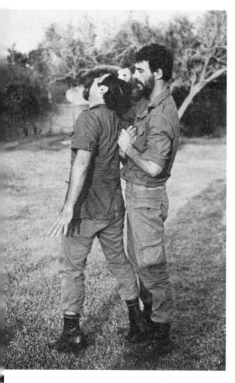

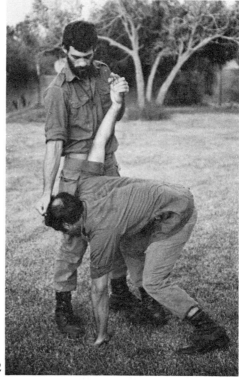

2

3. Prisoner falls onto left side and shifts left foot behind captor's left leg. He kicks captor's shin or knee with right foot.
4. Prisoner pushes captor's left leg with his right leg and knocks him down.

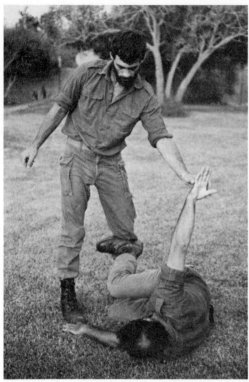

3

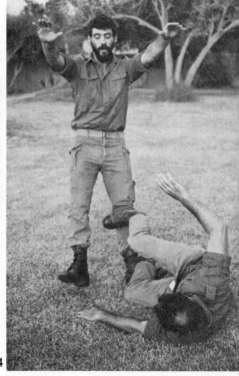

4

Self-Defense for Women— Special Advice

A WOMAN'S PHYSICAL STRENGTH is about two-thirds that of a man's, but woman is just as aggressive by nature. It is her traditional upbringing that puts a premium on her delicacy. "A woman's strength lies in her weakness" is an aphorism that loses its appeal when a woman is being attacked.

Remember: You have the power and the ability to overcome almost any attacker. You can rely on your own strength and on self-defense techniques to get you out of difficult situations. You must learn to overcome your embarrassment or discomfort when pushing off an attacker or a man who won't leave you alone. Generally, the sooner you ward off an attacker, the better your chances are of escaping unharmed. DON'T BE PASSIVE. Try to protect yourself and keep up an effective defense until you can escape.

This section is designed to give you some practical advice on self-defense. Contact combat techniques have been adapted to attack situations in which you might suddenly find yourself, including an attempt in a moving vehicle. You don't have to be very strong to master these skills. Their purpose is to stun your attacker by striking the vulnerable parts of his body, regardless of how strong he is, to give you time to escape. They are easy to learn. Get to know the vulnerable parts of the body (see page 77), and familiarize yourself with the exercises. When you first begin to practice, concentrate on the correct execution of the movement itself. Work on accuracy next. Pick a spot on the wall and try to strike it consistently. Then increase your speed. Finally, practice your self-defense exercises with a partner.

Know-how, alertness and composure will help you out of unpleasant situations. We hope the exercises that follow will be useful in preventing attacks on women in general and on soldiers who hitchhike in particular.

The Attack Kick

Drive off your attacker *before* he gets a chance to grab you. The attack kick lets you aim at the attacker's groin from a safe distance.

Take one step forward. Lean back, throw your other leg up. Be sure to raise your knee high. Kick hard. Delivered correctly, this kick will immobilize the attacker.

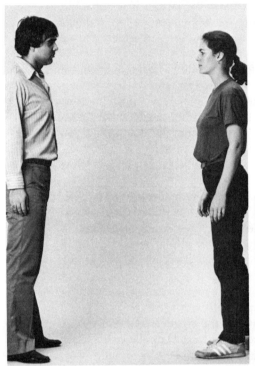

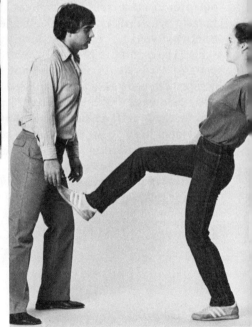

Elbow Blow

You are walking down the street, when someone grabs your arm from behind. Use the momentum, and step back and pivot on the foot on the same side as the arm that is grabbed. Push off on the opposite foot and strike a blow to the attacker's chin with your elbow.

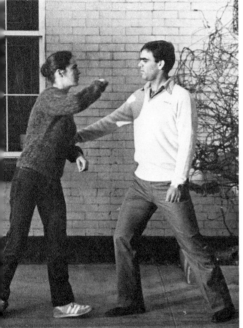

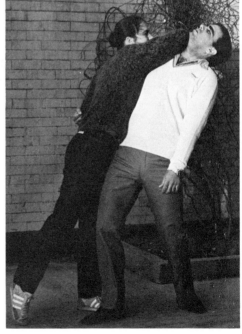

Breaking Free from an Open Front-Hold

You are grabbed from the front but your arms are free. Break loose by directing a knee kick at the attacker's groin. Lean forward and quickly draw your leg up.

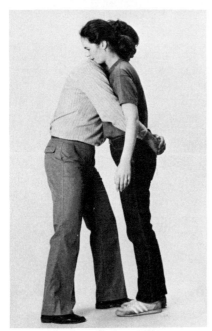

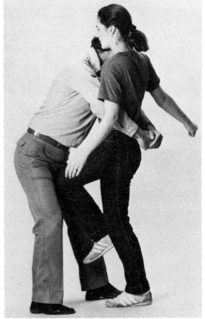

Breaking Free from a Closed Front-Hold

You are grabbed from the front and your arms are pinned beneath your attacker's. Move your hips back, reach down, and direct a finger jab to his groin.

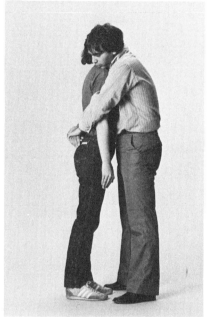

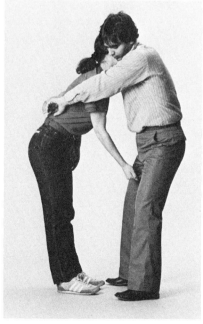

Breaking Free from a Closed Back-Hold

An attacker grabs you from behind, your arms are pinned beneath his. Lean forward and hit him hard in the groin with your fist or extended fingers. Or, lean forward and kick him hard in the shin with your heel, then stomp on his foot. (See next exercise.)

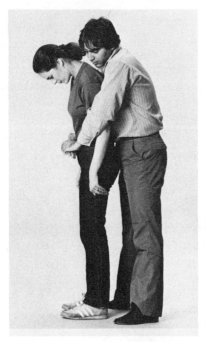

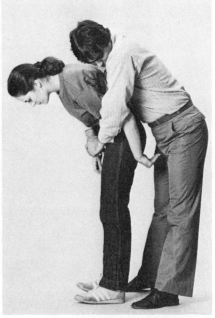

Breaking Free from an Open Back-Hold

An attacker grabs you from behind, but your arms are free. Grip one of his fingers in two hands, and bend it back as far as you can. At the same time, bend forward until you are looking between his legs. Kick him hard in the shin with your heel, then stomp on his foot with your heel.

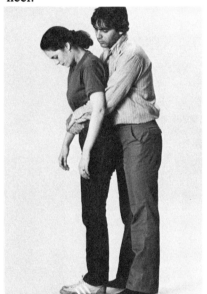
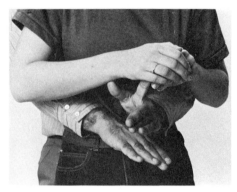
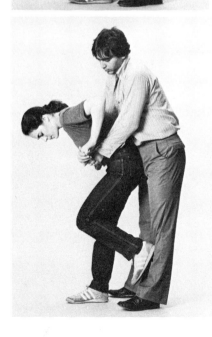
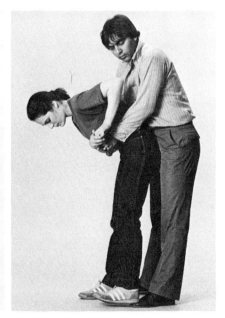

Or, use the full force of your body to swing around and strike backward with your elbow. Aim at his neck and head.

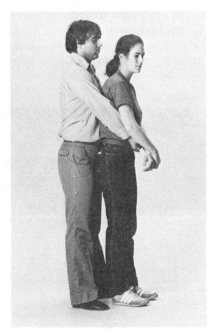

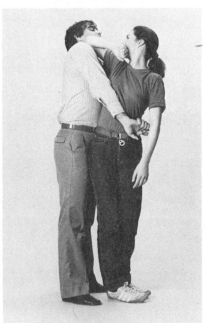

Breaking Free in a Car

When you hitchhike, you may meet an aggressive driver who has his own ways of getting you to pay for the ride. When you first get into the car, take a look around. Where is the door handle? Where are the locks? Are they electronic? Where are the controls? How much room do you have?

If you've had the misfortune of meeting up with a driver who likes to get cozy with women, make it quite clear to him that being a woman does *not* make you weaker. Stay calm. Try not to let your concern show. If he starts making friendly offers, reply quietly but firmly. In most cases he will instantly take a renewed interest in the road. But he may refuse to take a hint.

Let's say the driver grabs you as you are trying to get the door open and he pulls you toward him. You have several options:

1. BACKWARD ELBOW BLOW

Instead of resisting the attacker's pull on your arm, make use of the momentum. Swing around and plant your left elbow on his chin or throat.

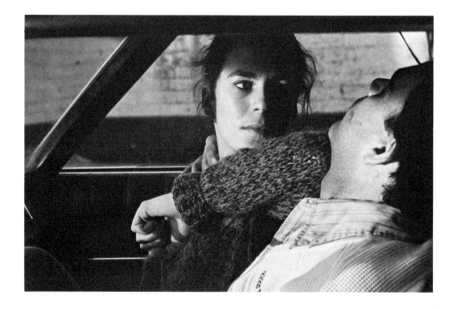

2. FINGERS IN THE EYES

With fingers extended, swing your right hand up and jab the attacker's eyes with full force. The attacker will suffer a temporary loss of vision and will reach up to protect his eyes, leaving his body vulnerable to further blows, if necessary.

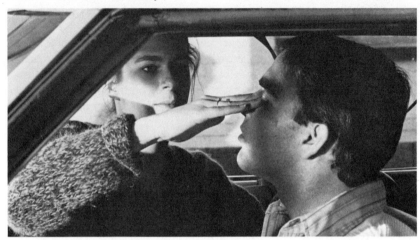

3. HEEL OF HAND TO BASE OF NOSE

As the attacker grabs your left arm, swing around and strike him at the base of his nose with the heel of your right hand, hard enough to push his head back.

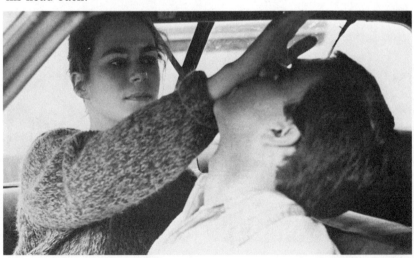

Breaking Free When Lying on the Ground

If you've been forced to the ground on your back, you are at a disadvantage. But you can break loose. Push the attacker upward and forward by raising your pelvis off the ground. At the same time, raise your arms and push his arms straight over your head. The attacker will naturally put his hands forward to block his fall. Before he falls, quickly

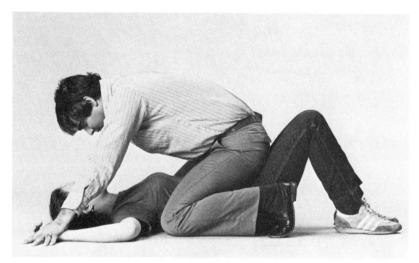

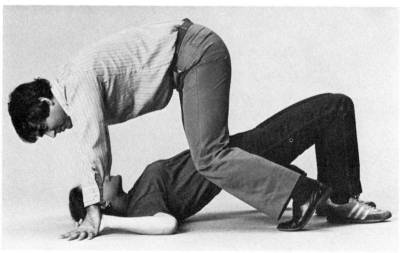

clench your fist and hit him in the groin. This blow will push him off you and let you get up and escape.

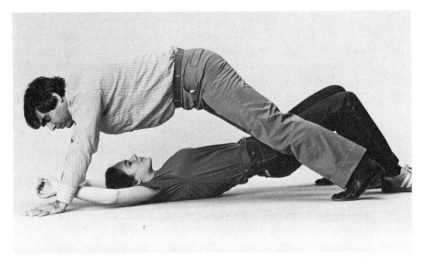

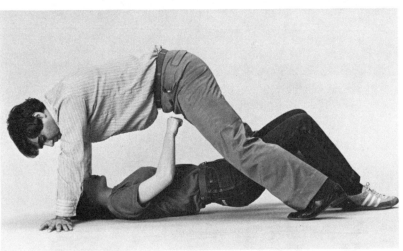

PART III

Obstacles

How to Overcome Obstacles

THE I.D.F. HAS DEVELOPED obstacle-crossing techniques that are highly efficient and effective, but are not necessarily the ones a person would naturally resort to. To improve performance, there is a need for explanation, instruction, and changes in natural locomotor patterns that require skill and practice.

This chapter covers different obstacle-crossing techniques and offers illustrations of how they are performed in the I.D.F. They can easily be adapted for civilian use. We also offer a few lessons as examples of the training program and the points to be emphasized. We hope you will succeed in applying these tips for your own uses or for the use of your trainees whenever the need arises.

Exercise 1 Hand and Foot Beam

Description of the obstacle: Round, horizontal beam, perpendicular to course, 1 meter above ground
Length: 4 meters or more
Diameter: 20 centimeters

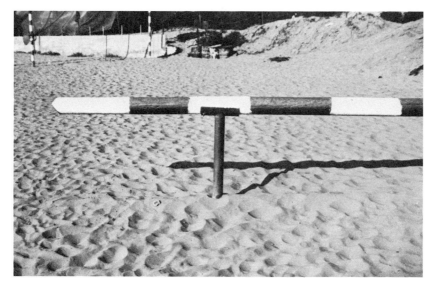

Similar objects in the terrain: Stone fences, tree trunks, low walls

Objective of training: Technique to scale a low (waist-high) obstacle (wall or fence)

Skills: Hand and foot crossing technique; coordination

Muscles that are especially active: Thighs, forearms, hips

Performance technique:
1. Run to obstacle, place left hand on beam, slightly bent, palm forward. Spring off left foot, straighten right leg and place inner ridge of shoe heel on beam.

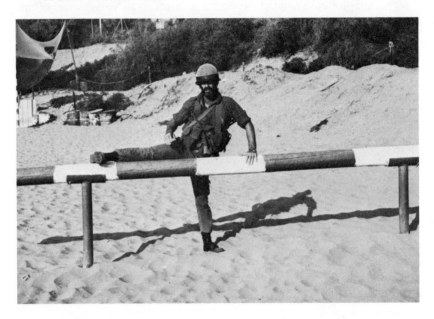

2. Straighten left arm, lifting body up, and pass left leg between beam and right leg.

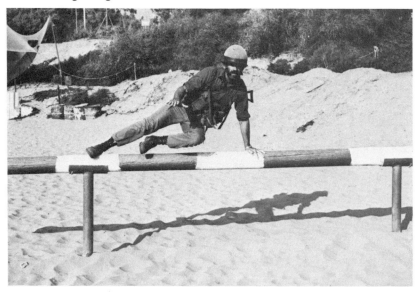

3. Land on left leg, push off beam with left hand and continue running.

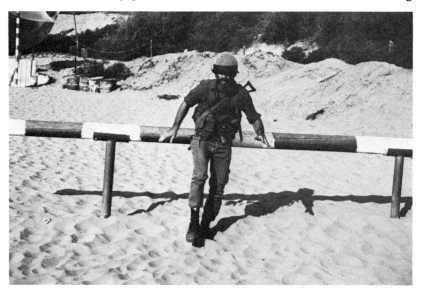

Points to emphasize: Keep body low to ground by leaning toward beam while running.

Exercise 2 Horizontal Ladder

Description of the obstacle: Iron ladder, 40 centimeters between rungs
Height: 2.5 meters
Width: 1 meter
Length: 4 meters

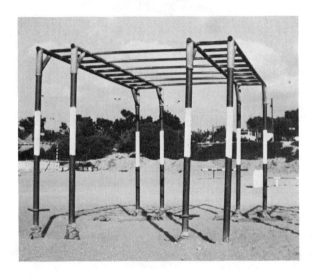

Similar objects in the terrain: A water pipe or beam suspended over an obstacle

Objective of training: Technique to clear obstacles that cannot be crossed on foot, using arms and hands only

Skills: Advancing while hanging from hands; coordination.

Muscles that are especially active: Arms, elbows, hands, and shoulders

Performance technique:
 1. *Forward movement*
    a. Run to obstacle, leap and grab first rung in overhand grip (palms forward).
    b. Advance by moving hands one after the other, alternating bars with each hand and swinging from side to side to the end of the obstacle.
    c. Release hands, drop to ground, and continue running.

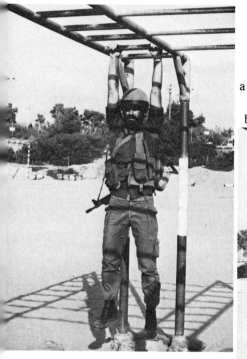

a

b

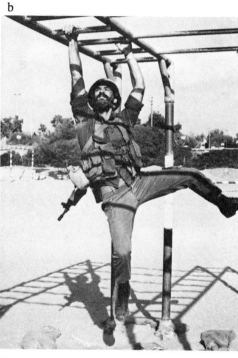

c

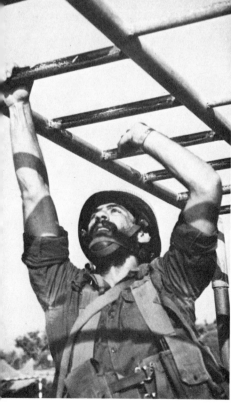

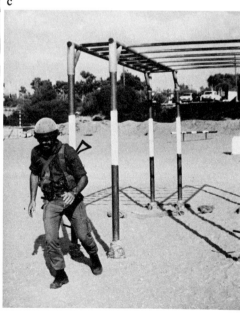

2. *Lateral movement*
   a. Run to obstacle and leap and grab side of ladder in overhand grip (palms forward).
   b. Advance by sliding hand away and bringing other hand to first, with legs swinging freely. Release grip, drop to the ground, make a quarter turn to left, and continue running.

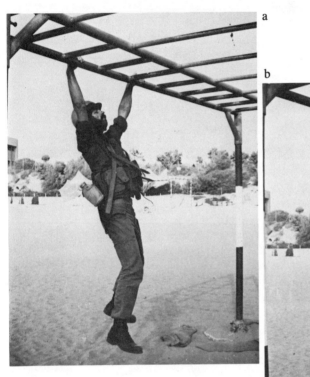
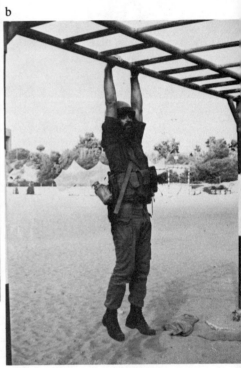

Points to emphasize:

1. Swing body forward when moving the first hand. Swings should not be severe or wild, but enough to give you momentum and help you move your hands.
2. As hand moves out, open legs. As the other hand moves to join first hand, close legs.

Exercise 3 Medium-High Wall

Description of the obstacle: Concrete wall
Height: 180 centimeters
Length: 4 meters or more
Width: 20 centimeters

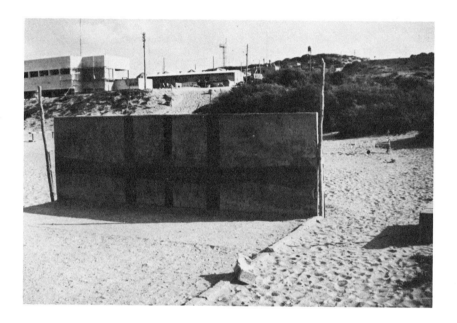

Similar objects in the terrain: Walls around yards and homes, high fences

Objective of training: Techniques to scale medium-high walls

Skills: Coordination; climbing ability

Muscles that are especially active: Knees, arms and thighs

Performance technique:

1. Run to wall, leap off left foot, place right foot on wall, straighten right leg to thrust body upward and grab top of wall.

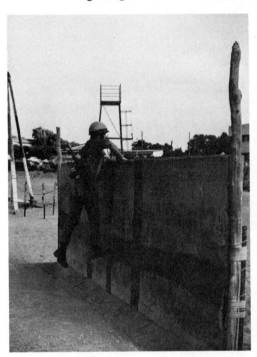 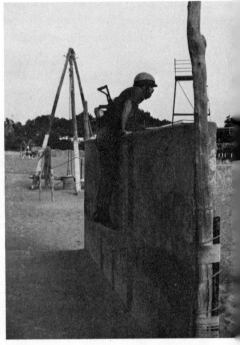

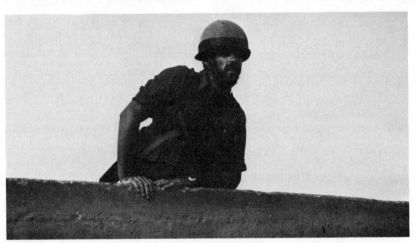

2. Place left forearm on top of wall (90-degree angle at elbow). Set right palm on top of wall, fingers pointed in the direction of movement. Lean hand and body forward from waist.

3. Raise left leg, straighten and extend to the side from hip until it rests on top of wall.

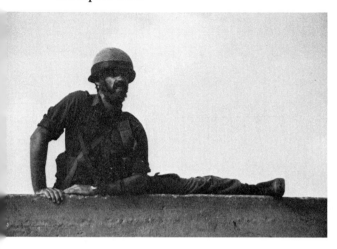

4. Lean body forward from waist. Bring left arm over wall, palm flat against wall for support. Right arm stays as it was. Bring right leg up to left leg.

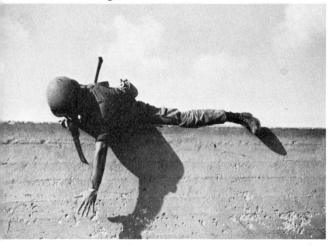

5. With right hand and left leg, raise body high enough to bring right leg and body over wall, but no higher. Push off the wall with both hands for side landing on feet.
6. Continue running.

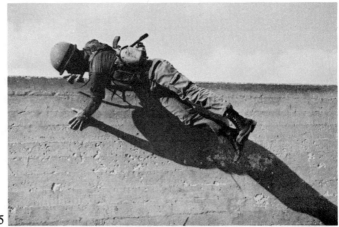

5

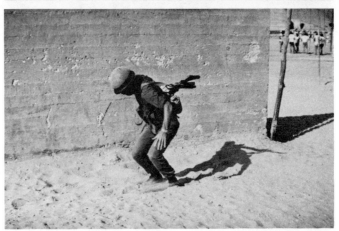

6

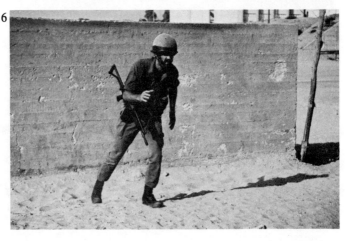

Exercise 4 Rope Climbing

Description of the obstacle: Six-meter-long rope, 18 mm. thick, suspended from a beam 3.5 meters above the ground

Similar objects in the terrain: Ropes used to climb high walls or embankments

Objective of training: Use of rope for getting over high obstacles

Skills: Rope-climbing technique; coordination

Muscles that are especially active: Shoulders, arms, hands, chest, lower abdomen, thighs, knees

Performance technique:
1. With rope dangling between legs, grip with both hands, one at chest height and the other above the head. Lift right knee (or left if you prefer) and turn it out, so that rope falls across ankle to the outside of foot.

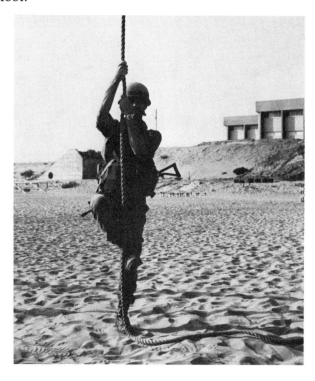

2. Lift body off ground; gather rope with left foot so that rope loops under right boot and over left boot, passing through arch.
3. Tighten rope around shoes. Left leg is vertical and right leg horizontal. Left foot tightens the rope to the inner, horizontal edge of the right boot. The angle between knees is 90 degrees. Body weight shifts to right foot to increase pressure on the rope. By gripping the rope with his feet, the climber "breaks" it at two points, thus increasing the friction and diminishing the chances of sliding down.

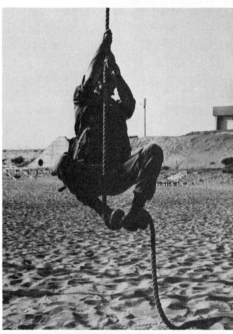

2

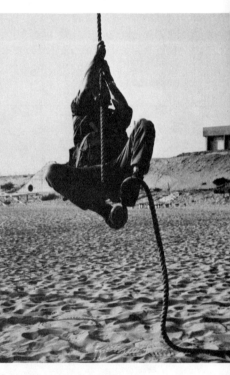

3

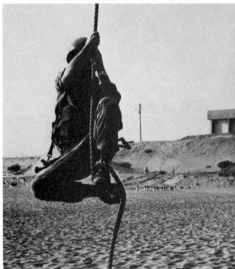

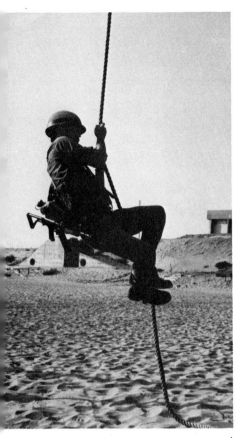

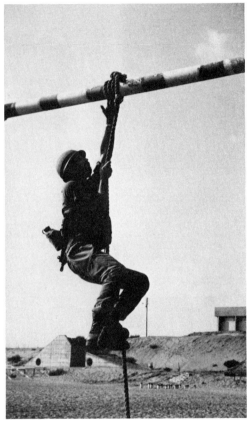

4

4. Straighten knees, move hands higher up on rope, move up another step and continue until hand touches upper beam. Use the leg muscles only. The hands support the body at chest level. The legs are lifted to the next step by the contraction of the abdominal muscles and thigh flexors.
5. Descend by jumping or by applying the same step-by-step procedures in reverse. Land and continue running. Repeat this entire sequence until ready to land softly to the ground. If possible, avoid sliding down; the friction is likely to cause rope burns to the hands.

PART IV

Physiological Aspects of Physical Effort

Introduction

THE WARM-UP

THE WARM-UP PREPARES the muscles and joints and the circulatory and respiratory systems for the coming efforts. Without proper warm-up, muscles, joints and ligaments may be too tight, and injury could result. The warm-up also increases respiration and circulation so that muscles can work aerobically—that is, they draw energy from the increased oxygen in the bloodstream, rather than from themselves. Unless you reach the aerobic level before strenuous exercise begins, you won't be able to perform at your maximum ability.

Proper warm-up usually takes from 5 to 10 minutes. The exercises on pages 24 and 34, and jogging at an easy pace for 400 meters, should be part of your warm-up routine. You'll know you're sufficiently warmed up when you work up a light sweat, your range of movement is increased, and your breathing is comfortable. You should feel as though you'd be able to run for a long time.

THE COOL-DOWN

The cool-down is as important as the warm-up. The active muscles become shortened and tense during strenuous effort. They must be restored to their normal length (stretching the shortened muscle while contracting the longer muscle). while the circulation of oxygen-saturated blood is decreased, and the accumulation of lactic acid in muscles, which causes cramps, is prevented. Exercises, such as those on pages 27 and 53, performed at an easy pace, can be used to cool down. Walking also helps relax the active muscles. After the cool-down, relax completely by lying down and breathing deeply.

GENERAL

A. Physical activity involves an element of risk, especially for those over 35 who have taken up the challenge of a physical fitness program after a prolonged period of inactivity.

213

B. Excess activity can cause injuries. Have a thorough physical examination and discuss your planned program with your doctor *before* you begin. Start at the minimum level or lower, gradually and slowly working up to your desired level of fitness. Learn to perform the exercise correctly.

THE EFFECTS OF PHYSICAL EXERTION ON SYSTEMS IN THE BODY

Several systems of the body work at an accelerated pace when physical activity is increased. The greater the exertion, the harder they work. If the systems are in any way deficient, the additional stress can be dangerous.

The Circulatory System

THE HEART

The heart pumps blood, the carrier of oxygen and energy, through the cardiovascular system. As the amount of energy needed for physical activity increases, the heart must work harder. The incredible complexity of this mechanism, with its network of chambers and valves operating in perfect coordination, makes it vulnerable to certain afflictions:

1. Athlete's Heart. Physical exertion strengthens and enlarges the heart as it does any other muscle. The symptoms of athlete's heart—lowered pulse (60 beats per minute), irregular heartbeat, and changes in the EKG similar to those associated with certain heart conditions, which may mislead the attending physician—are especially prevalent among people who participate in regular, rigorous fitness programs. Heart enlargement usually subsides as soon as the level of physical activity is reduced.

As a rule, athlete's heart is not dangerous, so long as the enlargement of the heart is not out of proportion. Occasionally, however, athlete's heart syndrome may occur. Athletes who put an unrelenting and very intense strain on their heart and respiratory system may be afflicted with accelerated pulse, weakness, chest pains, shortness of breath and even some irregularities in the working of the heart. These factors have the cumulative effect of lowering overall physical fitness. The solution lies in prolonged rest and a change in training programs. This is one of the reasons for taking an EKG before starting any intensive physical fitness program and repeating the test annually.

2. Exertion Syndrome. The symptoms of exertion syndrome are similar to those of chronic athlete's heart: rapid heartbeat (tachycardia), flushed face, shortness of breath and fatigue. But they develop entirely differently. Exertion syndrome appears whenever the body is under physical stress. It occurs most frequently in people who have not been active for a length of time, e.g., high school graduates who are not accustomed to the physical exertion required during military training.

Exertion syndrome should not be viewed as a disease, but as a condition produced by prolonged inactivity that can be rectified by a gradual, regular and regimented program of physical training. In studies conducted for the I.D.F., soldiers who had suffered from this syndrome and had been classified as physically inadequate by military standards scored a marked improvement in their physical condition after regular participation in a physical training program, and were eventually even assigned to combat units. This change also improved the trainees' self-confidence and self-image.

3. Heart Diseases. A heart attack is a severe occurrence; it may damage an essential, life-supporting system. It is a condition most likely to occur in certain age groups: men over 40 and women over 50. It does, however, also occur among younger people. In its broadest sense, the heart attack comprises several diseases:

a. ANGINA PECTORIS arises from arteriosclerosis. The blood vessels that lead to the heart are gradually narrowed by the deposit of cholesterol, lipids and calcium on their walls. The narrowed vessels may be able to carry an adequate supply of blood to the heart during normal daily activity but may prove inadequate during physical exertion. Insufficient oxygen to the heart muscle produces acute pain in the chest area. As soon as the exertion is stopped, this pain may disappear or it may be relieved by nitroglycerin pills, which widen the blood vessels. Generally, those who suffer from angina should abstain from strenuous physical activity.

b. ARRHYTHMIA is an irregularity of the heart's rhythm (faster or slower than normal, or uneven), caused by the release of chemical substances into the nervous system. The cause and the type of arrhythmia must first be diagnosed before a fitness program is undertaken. Some become more acute with physical effort, while others are actually relieved by exercise.

c. MYOCARDIAL INFARCTION occurs when a blood vessel is completely blocked, cutting off the blood supply to the heart muscle and causing residual damage. It may occur when a lipidic deposit of blood clot breaks free from the coronary wall and moves through the bloodstream until it becomes lodged in an artery. Symptoms include acute chest pains extending to the left arm and neck, accompanied by pallor and perspiration. A patient suffering from a myocardial infarction must be treated in a hospital as quickly as possible. Heart failure caused by myocardial infarction is usually sudden and unpredictable.

d. HEART MURMURS can be caused by a valve that does not close completely and allows blood to escape prematurely from one chamber to another, or by perforation of the septum. In acute valvular conditions, some degree of cardiac insufficiency will be present. Strenuous physical activity should be avoided. If the perforation in the septum is small (a less noticeable murmur), restriction of physical activity may not be necessary, although there should be regular medical supervision.

Exertion can aggravate or improve heart conditions and it is this duality that fuels the dispute among doctors over the effects of physical activity, especially among those over 35. There are several predisposing factors in heart diseases: prolonged periods of physical inactivity, excessive smoking, a high-fat diet, hypertension, emotional stress and heredity. Research findings generally acknowledge:

1. Excessive and unusually intense physical effort by those over age 35 can be dangerous without the supervision of a doctor.
2. An overweight person who smokes heavily and spends most of his or her time behind a desk at emotionally taxing jobs ought to begin with only the mildest program of physical activity under medical supervision.
3. A person who engages in an ordered, regular fitness program may develop additional capillaries that would not develop in an inactive person. This system can become an effective bypass if the artery is blocked by a thrombosis (blood clot) and may thus reduce the severity of the disease. In addition, physical activity reduces the predisposing factors in heart attacks by promoting a healthy life-style and reducing emotional pressures.

The Vascular System

The vascular system carries the energy that the body requires for its work and gets rid of waste; the entire body depends on its smooth and efficient operation. The blood vessels constitute a closed system and the liquid within it is under different hydrostatic pressures at different points. Blood pressure is measured indirectly in the brachial artery (upper arm) using a sphygmomanometer connected to an inflatable cuff. Let us familiarize ourselves with a few terms, for a better understanding of this subject:

Systolic pressure (maximal) is the pressure of the blood forcing its way through the artery as the pressure in the cuff is released. Its normal value is 120 mm. Hg. (millimeters of mercury).

Diastolic pressure (minimal) is the pressure of the blood against the walls of the blood vessels with the final release of the cuff. It is normally about 80 mm. Hg. This difference of about 40 mm. Hg. between the systolic and the diastolic pressures is known as the pulse pressure.

The following are some of the factors that influence blood pressure:

The heart—The weaker it is, the lower the blood pressure.

Peripheral resistance—The larger the circumference of the blood vessels, the less resistance within the arterial walls to the passage of blood. The narrowing of the blood vessels, therefore, will result in increased blood pressure.

The quantity of blood—Injury that causes loss of blood will also reduce blood pressure.

Blood viscosity—Blood pressure increases in direct proportion to such factors as the quantity of the platelets.

Elasticity—The arteries can change their width as needed to regulate the pressure.

A blood pressure of 160/100 mm. Hg. is considered high and blood pressure under 90/60 is considered low.

Low blood pressure is manifested in weakness, a tendency to tire quickly, dizzy spells and fainting. High blood pressure (hypertension) results in dizziness, nausea, headaches, flushed face, bloodshot eyes, loss of consciousness and hemorrhages. Hypertension can create cerebral hemorrhages followed by a stroke and, in extreme cases, death. Since physical exertion causes blood pressure to rise, anyone with blood pressure higher than 160/100 mm. Hg. should consult his or her physician before starting any exercise program. After the blood pressure is brought under control with medication and lowered to acceptable levels, the prospective athlete may begin physical activity.

The Respiratory System

The role of the respiratory system is to supply oxygen and remove carbon dioxide from the blood.

A. There are two types of respiration:
   1. External—Air is taken into the lungs. The nose and windpipe take part in the external breathing process.
   2. Internal—Oxygen is transferred from the lungs to the blood and from the blood to the cells of the body.

B. Regulation and breathing under exertion

The body requires more oxygen during exertion than it does at rest. Sense receptors monitor carbon dioxide levels in the blood, and signal us to automatically draw a breath when we need more oxygen. During physical activity, the rate and depth of breathing accelerate. The untrained athlete tends to exaggerate the need for faster breathing. It is more important to relax, so that the depth of breathing is increased.

We can, of course, consciously control our breathing, but it should be limited to exhaling during exertion and inhaling during the less strenuous parts of the exercise.

C. Psychological effects

Physical exertion coupled with tension (e.g., during a physical fitness test) cause pulse and breathing rates to accelerate and perspiration to form, even before physical exertion begins. While these developments cause no physiological harm in themselves, they are liable to detract from the score if a low pulse rate is one of the criteria. Generally speaking, pulse and breathing rates adjust to physiological needs within a few minutes after the exertion begins.

D. The Valsalva phenomenon

Named after the doctor who first described its symptoms, the Valsalva phenomenon is characterized by a temporary cessation of the oxygen supply to the brain. The symptoms are dizziness, fainting or unconsciousness. It happens when an effort is made to exhale with great force but the air cannot escape because of a constriction of the throat, diaphragmatic, abdominal, or thoracic (chest) muscles. There is sudden pressure within the thoracic cavity, preventing the regular flow of blood to the heart and lungs. Cardiac strength and arterial pressure decline, depriving the tissues of oxygen. The brain is the first to be affected, and fainting results. In addition, the heart must compensate for the resistance in the narrowed blood vessels and overcome the deficient supply of oxygen to itself. This burden could prove detrimental even to a sound heart, let alone to a deficient one. The Valsalva phenomenon, in effect, forces the heart to work anaerobically until the oxygen supply is restored.

Many physical activities may place the body in a state that approximates the Valsalva syndrome—weight lifting, wrestling, isometric exercises, etc. Psychologically, you think you have to hold your breath when exerting yourself, but it's more effective to breathe regularly. Adverse symptoms can be avoided by correct breathing: exhaling during the most strenuous part of the activity, inhaling during the easy part.

The Muscular and Skeletal Systems

A. Muscular system

1. *Fatigue*

   A muscle's ability to contract is limited. Sooner or later, they tire out. Pain and heaviness result, forcing the athlete to cease the particular activity. He or she simply can't move another muscle.

   Muscle fatigue occurs in several ways:

   a. The body cannot supply the muscle with the energy it needs, as the consumption of energy becomes more rapid than its production.

   b. Fatigue of the nerves that transfer the stimuli to the muscle, following the depletion of the chemical that makes it possible for the stimulus from the nerve to reach the muscle. A tired muscle must be rested long enough to allow the body to replenish its energy supply, to get rid of the wastes and to facilitate the conduction of the stimuli from nerve to muscle.

2. *Aches*

   These result from strenuous exercise after prolonged inactivity. The aches begin after a day or two and last about six days. They are caused by the rupture of microscopic muscle fibers and/or the connective tissue between the muscle and the tendon. The fibers heal with rest and a decrease in the amount of physical activity. Aches can be avoided by beginning a fitness program slowly and working up to the desired fitness level gradually.

3. *Cramps*

   During prolonged exertion, the spaces in between the muscle fibers can fill with lactic acid and other waste, preventing proper contraction of the muscle. A forceful involuntary muscle contraction results, causing severe pain. Relief comes by stretching the muscle until the normal circulation of the blood can carry the waste away. Massage or hot water will help. This should be done immediately, to protect the muscle and to avoid rupture of the tendon from overextension. This is why gradual warm-up and cool-down are so important.

B. Skeletal system

1. *Backaches*

Backaches are among the most common affliction. The interver-
tebral cartilage of the spine, especially in the lumbar region
(lower back), may be damaged by a bad landing from a jump or
fall, incorrect lifting of a heavy weight, or other injury. Cartilage presses down on the nerve ends emerging from the spine
through the vertebral pores, causing sharp pain, which also radi-
ates to the lower limbs. This can require prolonged treatment or
hospitalization. Exercises on page 68 can strengthen the back
muscles and help hold the spine and cartilage in proper align-
ment.

2. *Walking (stress) fracture*

A stress fracture is a microscopic fracture of the bone, and most
often occurs in the shins, thighs and feet. Stress fractures are
usually experienced by soldiers of high motivation, who feel a
slight pain, but continue to train without seeking proper treatment. After a few weeks the pain becomes more severe, forcing
the soldier to see a doctor. But by then, the fracture has grown
and it takes longer to heal. It's caused most frequently by too
much effort without graduation.

If you feel undefined pain, go to a doctor. You may have a stress
fracture. Treatment is rest. It will heal itself.